"After working with persons with head injuries for the last twelve years, I have yet to hear what peoples' innermost thoughts were during their struggle to regain their identity, until now. Surviving Black Ice is an honest account of life after a head injury, and will be a great help to other survivors, family members and professionals."

Beth Edelberg-Cardillo, M.Ed., L.S.W.
Director, East Mountain Head Injury Center
Westfield, MA

"...Fierce's ability to turn this tragic occurrence into a triumph of human courage and strength is both encouraging and uplifting. . . I believe that projects such as Surviving Black Ice can help promote support of brain injury in the public, as well as offer both hope and optimism to people who have acquired a brain injury."

James S. Brady, Vice-Chairman
National Brain Injury Association
Washington, DC

"I found David's struggle in recovering from TBI to be inspirational; highlighting this most complex and all-encompassing process with candor and humor. . . I believe Surviving Black Ice is excellent and important, for other survivors as well as for all those who become part of the recovery process."

Glenn Fagen, Ph.D.
Neuro-psychologist,
Weldon Center for Rehabalitation
Springfield, MA

DAVID W. FIERCE

SURVIVING BLACK ICE

Published by Writer's Block Press

Writer's Block Press
P.O. Box 2456
Manchester CT 06045, USA

www.writersblockpress.com

First Writer's Block Press printing, March, 2002

Printed in the United States of America

Cover snowflake image used with permission:
Rasmussen & Libbrech, www.snowcrystals.net

In memory of Dennis

Acknowledgments

Many people have given their time and talent to help me bring this work to you. My thanks go to all the people at Saint Francis Medical Center who gave me the encouragement to begin putting my feelings and observations into writing. I am also greatly indebted to the Nasjleti's, David and Margot, for allowing me to benefit from their expertise—especially Margot.

Margot you inspired me to great heights, giving freely of your time and abilities, prodding me on, challenging me to be more than I am.

I need to thank Wayne Smith who, by his actions and wisdom, re-kindled my desire to put Black Ice in the public eye and, hopefully, help those in need.

And through it all, beginning to end, Lex Nasjleti.

Black Ice

Black Ice: slang noun, 1. A type of ice which crystallizes transparently as a result of dry climatic conditions, and is unseen. 2. An unseen impediment or condition which may propel an object in an undetermined direction or cause to lose directional control.

Introduction

I am among a relatively new breed of survivors. I have been told that until approximately ten years before my accident, people with similar types of head trauma did not survive. Apparently, at that time, drugs had been developed that reduced brain swelling. Before then, those with closed head injuries would always die. I want to use my story as a tool to encourage, enlighten, and give warning but also hope to so many people whose lives have been affected, either directly or indirectly, by brain damage.

This is not just a nice story about a miraculous recovery, it is the story of a struggle to survive and succeed. I strive to tell the story from my viewpoint alone, but with one exception: to detail the accident, I have had to use a factual framework that was told to me by others. I had many opportunities to receive input from my family because my mother and sister had written many things down, but I want to tell this story from my own memory and perspective.

My entire family and some of my friends went through terrible emotional trauma. I sometimes think I got the better part of this tragic period. Because of the great pain my family went through, I think failure to record my experience would be a great disservice. I can only hope this work reaches some of the growing number of family members, professionals, and other caregivers who have a relationship with someone who has sustained brain injury.

I offer some staggering statistics published by the National Brain Injury Foundation. As family members, professionals, and caregivers know, the following numbers are constantly rising.

- 2 million head injuries occur each year in the U.S.

- A head injury occurs every 15 seconds in this country.

- 75,000 - 100,000 Americans die each year as a result of traumatic head injury.

- 500,000 people each year will require hospitalization for traumatic head injuries.

- 70,000 - 90,000 individuals each year will suffer life long physical, intellectual, and psychological disabilities as a result of their head injuries.

- Tragically, two thirds of those who sustain head injuries are under the age of 34.

Although my condition was diagnosed as "Severe Closed Head Injury," the lessons I've learned, the feelings I've had, and the struggles I've had to overcome can be applied to many people in other circumstances. As you read the story of my recovery, you may notice similarities to someone close to you and come to understand their frustrations. In my attempt to portray the struggles, frustrations, and experiences I went through personally, it is my hope that I may shed some light on your own.

By taking you through ten years of my life, I am certain that significant others can gain an awareness and understanding of many basic realities of rehabilitation. I refer to anyone who has had some form of brain injury (head injury, stroke, brain tumor, aneurysm, or any other brain-damaging occurrence) as "survivor," and anyone who loves and cares for that injured person as "significant other." Starting with the first broken, vague memories I had and moving forward, I record my impressions from a survivor's perspective and make commentary about those experiences that seem to me to have contributed significantly to the progress of my healing and growth. I take the reader with me as I struggle though rehabilitation: hospitalization, outpatient therapy, marriage, relocation, employment, divorce, relationships, and higher education.

I have been told by so many people over the years to "write a book," but I think that choosing this time in my life, this point in my recovery, is crucial. I have allowed enough time to pass to reach a level of maturity that enables me to relay the lessons I've learned and the insights I've had in a sensible and discerning manner.

I was twenty-three years old when the accident occurred. I began writing this account shortly before the tenth anniversary of this tragic and wonderful incident, ten long years in which I have, almost literally, lived another lifetime, certainly another reality.

I admit to being human. Over the years, I have become tired of trying to overcome obstacles, tired of people accusing me of being drunk or high. I have become depressed, angry with God, ready to give up, willing to remain where I was—never to try and to fail at anything again. I even tried to take my own life. Gradually, I learned I will never be finished learning. There comes a certain peace of mind when you realize you will never "arrive." Peace comes when you admit that life is a process… one that will never be easy… for anybody.

I truly believe that together and as individuals, we are all here to learn, to develop, and to survive our own black ice.

August - 1996

Out of Nothing

Someone's pushing me in a wheelchair... past the nursing station [How I knew it was a nursing station I don't know.] ... *into the elevator. I think there are two people with me. We're going down. I think.*

We're going into a room with mats and bars. [I was only aware of the mats and the parallel bars. I know now it was a therapy room.] *They move my arms and legs around. I try to stand up and hold on with one arm to the parallel bars.* [I don't remember leaving that room.]

There's a Christmas tree by the nurses' station! I watch the lights as I sit in my wheelchair.

Here comes Lisa! No, her name is Brenda. She is leaving.

Oh, I love you! Whoever you are I need to kiss you!

I motion her to lean down. I grab her around the neck and kiss it feverishly. She's wearing something around her neck. I want her to take it off. My lips feel funny. It's hard to kiss.

[How I knew what it was like to kiss, I don't know. How I know it was love I felt, I don't know. It was more like a primordial longing for attention and affection. Kissing was difficult because the plastic surgeon had done massive reconstruction to my forehead, eyebrow, and mostly my upper lip. My lips were swollen. It was Brenda, and the "thing" around her neck was a neck-brace.]

She left. I think Mom's here. I think she's always here.

[I should have wondered what was going on, but I didn't. I didn't ponder my situation. I didn't consider my future or my past. I only thought about whatever was right in front of me. I simply reacted to people and stimuli. I didn't really think, contemplate, or regard anything.]

Now they are dressing me with real clothes and a coat! We go into different rooms and stop by a door to say good-bye. I guess I'm leaving. My Mom and some man are putting me into the back of a van. Everyone says "Good-bye." They're very nice. The man driving the van is nice. My Mom is here and Lynette. The way Lynette just takes charge of everything makes me feel safe.

[My sister Lynette is a beautiful, petite, 100 pound little fireball. The trauma and uncertainty of this event had put her into over-drive. She's a highly trained Critical Care Nurse. I couldn't have been in better care.]

Now they're taking me down the aisle of an airplane in a wheelchair. [I don't remember being in an airport or even being transferred from the van.] *Everyone is so nice. The flight seems so long. I smile, say things and people laugh.* [They were probably being more kind than I realized. I don't remember what I said, but I could only speak short, slurred sentences. The passengers probably did not even understand me, but they would laugh politely. I just remember being the center of attention.] *Lynette is taking control of everything and taking care of me. I feel really safe. She's a nurse! I feel really important. Finally… after forever… the plane is landing. They take me out of the seat and put me into a wheelchair. They're taking me off the plane. Everyone, the pilots, the stewardesses, they all stand at the door of the plane and wave goodbye... some of them are crying. I feel really sad.*

I'm being put into a car. Phil! My brother-in-law is driving! I think he is so cool. My sister and my brother-in-law! This is so great!

[I still didn't know or wonder about what was going on. Lynette later told me I tried to open the door while we were driving. I don't remember.]

Now I'm in a hospital bed. Something hurts down there. I keep telling them and rubbing... no one cares. [Later I learned my catheter was positioned incorrectly, and I was having a reaction.] *I'm in a big room. I know its Saint Francis Medical Center in Peoria, near my hometown.* [I remember being told which hospital I would be sent to while I was still in Colorado.]

What's going on? Why am I here? ... I know what happened... but why? How come I can't?... Was it my fault?... They say no, but was it? Mo was with me... How's Mo... How's Brenda? Was I driving? I'm so tired... can I just go to sleep now? I know these people... I remember this... I know I'm home... but I guess I'm safe... I see familiar things, but I'm not familiar; I'm different now.

I don't remember being told I was in an accident. My mother says she had explained my situation to me while I was in a coma and patiently continued to do so, as I became aware.

Now my memories are a mixture of personal experiences and the stories told to me. I am glad I waited as long as I did to record these happenings, for many reasons, mostly because now I am capable of understanding and communicating them. I also see that this story will have a happy ending.

The Journey of 10,000 Miles Begins

I have no recollection of the accident. I can remember a few things about the sunny, clear morning earlier, but most of that day and the weeks to come are a total blank. I only know stories I have been told and the results of an investigation that was done for legal reasons. My recollections may not be precisely factual, but my feelings, my analysis of those feelings, and my ability to communicate them are what matter. Many of the details are still unclear to me, but one thing is sure: I was not meant to die that day.

On November 8, 1984, I was driving with two friends from Colorado Springs to Denver by way of back roads. Somewhere near Salida, on a mountain pass, as an abrupt blizzard broke out, I came off a curve and hit a patch of black ice. When the car started to slide off the side of the mountain, I was able to pull it back on the road, but I had swerved the car into the opposite lane, into oncoming traffic.

I imagine the pick-up truck coming toward me hit the same patch of ice, and we collided head-on. I was not wearing a seat belt and slammed into the windshield. A year and a half after the accident, I talked to the State Trooper who came to the scene. "Normally," he said, "I would have ticketed you for not wearing a seat belt, but I was sure that you would not survive."

The driver of the pick-up, however, was wearing his seat belt. He was treated for a broken collarbone and released. The driver of the vehicle directly behind the man I hit was an ex-patrolman and paramedic from Alaska, someone trained in wintry highway emergency situations. He immediately removed me from the car, treated me for shock and stabilized me the best he could. After a 30 minute trip to a small hospital in Salida by ambulance, where I was stabilized further, a Life Flight helicopter from Colorado Springs arrived. They strapped me in and took-off.

When we finally arrived at Saint Francis Hospital in Colorado Springs, the pilot was unable to land because of cloud cover. A return to Salida seemed imminent. The moment before the pilot started to turn back… a hole in the clouds appeared! We landed and I was rushed directly to the operating room for surgery on my face and an exploratory laparotory.

Several days later, after the physicians were relatively certain I would survive, a feeding tube was inserted into my stomach, and I was given a tracheostomy to facilitate breathing with a respirator. My scalp had been torn away above my right eye exposing my skull; my right eye had been pulled from its socket; my right eyebrow was hanging by a few slim hairs; I had stuck my teeth through my upper lip almost tearing it completely off, and I had cracked my ribs and pelvis. Now when I reflect upon the injuries I sustained, I am thankful I was comatose, unable to feel pain consciously. At St. Francis, I was officially diagnosed: "Severe Closed Head Injury."

By this time, back in Illinois, my family had been contacted. A State Trooper called my father at work and told him his son had been killed in an auto accident. Someone told my mother that her son had been badly injured. My father did not tell her what he was told, thinking he'd spare my mother the shock. My entire family, my mom, dad, older sister, Lynette, and my younger brother, Daniel, were in Colorado Springs the next day. When they arrived at the hospital, they were taken into a room to be prepared for what they were about to see. My mother has told me that when they first stood beside my bed in Intensive Care, they beheld a sight so totally foreign, she felt she would be sick.

My scalp and right eye were completely covered with bandages. Everything above my neck was swollen beyond proportion. The right corner of my mouth was disproportionately lopsided with many sutures in it. Tubes had been stuck into me, and one was shoved down my throat. As they stood there in the silence of shock, the only sound was the rhythmic pumping of the respirator. I lay there unconscious, moving my legs about, sometimes thrashing them against the bed rails. They stood there speechless. My mother knew I must certainly be in extreme pain. Was this her son, was this her little boy?

My father stood in silent disbelief. According to my sister, his defense mechanism for this horror was denial. He maintained I'd pull through: this condition was only temporary. Maybe he was in denial, but I'd like to think he was voicing an affirmation of hope.

After a few days, my father and sister returned home to work. My brother went back to college. With arrangements made by the pastor of my parents' Mennonite church, my mom was able to stay with a Mennonite family. They let her borrow their four-wheel drive to visit me every day.

I remained in a coma for four weeks. During that time I had terrible seizures, my right eye would not close, I was fed through a feeding tube in my stomach, I breathed with the help of a machine, and I was contracting into a fetal position. I was paralyzed from head to foot, but just on my right side.

While I was in the coma, I developed pneumonia, which is quite common for patients in a coma and on respirators. When my right lung collapsed, alarms went off as I slipped into respiratory distress. However, a small metal tube, aptly named a chest tube, happened to be lying on a nearby tray when a physician happened to be checking on me. The doctor picked up the chest tube and stuck it through my ribs and into my lung, re-inflating it within seconds. It was as though he'd been there just waiting for the emergency to happen. After four weeks I came out of the coma… sort of.

One of the most frequent questions I hear is: "What was it like coming out of a coma?" I want to answer that question. By saying that I "sort of" came out of the coma, I mean that after four weeks I was no longer in a comatose state. Yet my mother said that for the next two weeks all I did was sleep and look around. In my case the best way to describe coming out of a coma is this: I don't know. It's like being born, I guess. Do you remember when you were born? When I awoke from the coma, I was like a newborn. I had no cognitive abilities, very simple thinking processes, and no ability to communicate. I had no connected thoughts. Simple words or phrases would come to mind with almost no logical patterns. I now remember these hospital scenes in glimpses, the same way someone remembers his first thoughts of childhood. My sister, Lynette, has said many times, "It was just like having a baby in the family."

Many people are curious about whether or not I could hear talking or remember being in a coma. This is the second most frequently asked question I receive. I think that the answer, as well as the answer to the previous question, is based upon the individual case. I can't remember hearing anything. If I took a trip down a tunnel or spoke with God, I don't remember. I was in a coma because my brain had been injured. Even if I had heard people speaking, I don't know that I would have been able to understand what was said. If it is true that an unborn child can receive stimulus by being spoken to in the womb, then maybe I did receive something.

I could tell more of the stories told to me about my stay in Colorado, but I want to emphasize what I can remember. I want to give an account from the perspective of a severely brain-injured survivor whose hidden stamina is driving him down the road of endless possibility. I have only used some of what I have been told to set the stage for this story. I hope that my experiences show that recovery is a painstaking, sometimes tedious process.

Recovery is *never* instantaneous… but it *always* seems miraculous!

Back to the Basics

Here I am. Back in Peoria. Home! I'm in a great big room that has a bed in each corner. They wake me up so early all the time. They take me out of bed. They put me in a wheelchair. They take me down the hall and give me showers. You can sit down in this shower. I brush my own teeth every morning but I can't use my right hand. I comb my own hair, but even when I put the comb in my right hand, I can't lift it up so high. It moves now, but not very good. I'm always so tired and they make me stay in that stinkin' wheelchair! Why won't they let me go back to bed? Every time someone walks by I ask so nice. I always say please. But no one will help me. I'm so tired; I just want to go to sleep. I just sit here and look around, listening, hoping for someone to be kind enough to me... to put me back in bed!

[I later learned I had to sit up for as long as I could to get used to being in an upright position.]

My aunt and uncle from Chicago are here! And they're here with my cousins... to see me! They all stand around while I sit in my *wheelchair. They just keep talking, moving around, asking me questions, and keep moving around. They just keep saying how good I'm doing and how lucky I am! Everyone says that I'm so lucky. Wow... really... I hope **you're** this lucky someday.*

I've recalled this event several times. I distinctly remember feeling sarcastic! I've decided I must have picked up that little bit of attitude from someone else. Maybe somebody who came to see me, trying to lighten the atmosphere, had said something to that effect. Looking back, I see the fact that I could recognize the sarcasm as significant: my thinking processes were already starting to improve. I'm sure I must have gotten it elsewhere because, in the first few months of my recovery, I had absolutely no original ideas and positively no sense of humor. I could not formulate my thoughts or speak quickly enough to be even remotely humorous. Comments I did make were very short, to the point, sometimes blunt, and always very literal. I lacked any spontaneity of expression and was chained to the sluggishness of both my physical and mental reaction time. I felt like I was trying to live my entire life in very thick syrup. Thoughts, speech, and movements came very slowly.

I feel funny. I really want to go back to sleep. I need to leave now. Please... I'm sorry... I know you've come a long way, but I feel really funny.

[I tried with my one good arm to wheel my chair away. I suddenly needed to be alone.]

I later understood that I could not yet filter out any stimuli. When anything was going on around me, I picked it all up with equal intensity whether or not the conversation was directed at me. I received everything. My visitors did not even talk to me much, but just listening to them talk to each other overwhelmed me. My reflective thinking and information processing ability had become damaged. I was, for all practical and relational purposes, a child again. I thought with the simple, selfish, egotistical mind of a child. Without malice or intent, I felt like the world revolved around my needs and me. Food and sleep consumed my thoughts. My room and the rehabilitation unit were my entire world.

After I had settled in my room, my physiatrist, Dr. Thomas Szymke, evaluated my condition. Only months later did I find out that Dr. Szymke had a conference with my parents and sister after the evaluation. He told them he had assessed me at the mental age of 9-10 months. They should not expect me ever to reach more than 18 months to 2 years mentally. Obviously this news devastated my parents.

Lynette later told me she almost jumped out of her chair to stand and argue with Dr. Szymke because she was sure there was a better prognosis. I don't know if Dr. Szymke's bedside manner was lacking or not, but his conclusion seems a little extreme. However, in the months to come, his skepticism about my progress, his sometimes blunt reactions, and his uncertainty about my abilities were just the therapy I required to progress further and further. It became a love/hate relationship in which I thought—*He says I can't? I'll show him!* In spite of his skepticism, I began therapy.

Although I had slept through Thanksgiving, my entire family brought Christmas to my room. I don't remember many of the details of my Christmas party at my new home, but I remember the love and patience I received. I can also remember my family remarking over and over about how well I was doing. My movements excited them as the paralysis was loosening its deadening hold on me, and I could now slur out an entire sentence with the best of them! Within just over a month I went from not knowing or thinking about what was happening to being aware of myself, to being aware of others.

God, I just move and slur through these stupid comments and they love it!

I felt so supported and accepted! It was the childhood I had never had. With no intentional manipulation, but with a child-like response to the reactions around me, I knew I could win praise and attention with every little bit of progress.

My family tells me they had to learn to be thankful for the small accomplishments. This appreciation and excitement over every little success made me try even harder. Some time later when I started moving my right side again, I thought I would try to open my own milk carton. It was dinner time and all my family had gathered around my bed. The head of my bed was elevated with my tray in front of me. I clumsily grabbed the top of the carton and struggled to pull the flaps apart.

God! What are they using for glue on these things these days!

My right hand was so weak that, as I pulled on one side of the flaps with my left hand, I just pulled the carton out of my right hand. Finally, I was able to hold the carton down on the tray with my right hand and tear open the flaps with my left. It wasn't pretty, but I had done it, and I had only spilled a little. My whole family applauded as though I had just finished a beautiful sculpture.

My mother had listened to the physicians who had told her to use any means to stimulate my mind. She brought in different objects to jog my memory and help in any way to rehabilitate me, showing me pictures of myself with friends and family or giving me a child's erasable sketch board to practice writing my name.

My family was always there. Somebody I knew always seemed to be around. I especially looked forward to the evenings when Phil, my brother-in-law, would visit. He and my sister started dating when I was a teenager, and I idolized him. Phil was a mechanic, so I had become a mechanic because of his influence in my life. Since my mind was maturing at a phenom-enal rate, I would become inquisitive about different topics and ask Phil's opinion. He was always willing to talk, no matter how sensitive or basic the subject. His eagerness to help in any way he could made me feel so important. I respected Phil.

My brother-in-law took an active role in my rehabilitation. He was always coming in with suggestions. I remember one time Phil brought in a racquetball I could squeeze to get stronger.

While I was in the hospital, I aged perhaps eight years intellectually and twelve years socially and emotionally. Like all adolescent young men, I started to think about sex. I recall one particular night in the hospital. As I lay in bed pondering the topic one evening, like so many things, I could remember the mechanics of sex, but the subtleties of it seemed vague. I felt just like a 6th grader who had heard or read how it was accomplished but didn't know the art of it.

The following evening, at the first opportunity, I leaned over to Phil and stammered—*Phil... I just can't seem to remember... you know... about sex.* Phil roared like a lion! He must have laughed for five minutes. Thank goodness no one else in my family was in the room at that moment for I'm sure they would have wanted to know what was going on. When he finally stopped, he sputtered, "Don't worry. It's like riding a bike! Some things will just come back to you!"

The Right to be Wrong

After Christmas another important person joined the group of visitors. Brenda, one of the two passengers in the car when the accident occurred, had recovered sufficiently from her own injuries to come to Peoria from her little hometown in South Dakota to rekindle the flames of the relationship I had rejected just weeks before the accident.

Brenda and I had met while I was living in Florida. She was vacationing there on Spring Break, and we had spent a few days together at the end of her vacation. After she returned to her home in South Dakota, we spent hours on the phone.

After two or three months, Brenda decided to move to Daytona Beach to live with me. However, the romantic scene that I had envisioned never materialized. When she arrived in Florida, she seemed like a total alien. She behaved in a way that was the complete opposite of her phone character.

I was excited, nervous, and apprehensive. This beautiful, simple, small town girl, who had swept me off my feet during her vacation, was coming to live with me! I was embarrassed by the fact that I was a dirty mechanic. I thought I needed a job that was more impressive. During the months prior to Brenda's arrival, I had enrolled in night school to get my real estate sales agent license. I started selling time-shares just a week before she arrived. Selling time-shares wasn't more impressive, but at least it was clean.

I had a new job, high hopes, and a new apartment for Brenda to live in; she entered with family problems, a load of doubt, a recently shattered romance, and an inexplicable, unwarranted coolness towards me. Brenda's arrival created an unexpected condition. It caused me to loose my bearings and to slide unpredictably out of control. Sound like black ice?

After a month of torment and indecision about my relationship with Brenda, I accepted the offer of a job selling time-shares at a mountainside ranch in Colorado. When I told Brenda I had accepted the position as assistant sales manager in Colorado and was leaving, I suggested that she return to South Dakota, but she wanted to come with me. I was excited by the idea because I thought that maybe, in a new environment, things would be different. But unfortunately the new surroundings did not mend the emotional wounds that I had already sustained. Only a week before the accident, I was trying to break off my relationship with Brenda. The relationship had become far too complicated and emotionally exhausting.

I was caught up in the time-share sales life-style: fast-paced and nomadic. Sales at the ranch weren't going as successfully as I had expected, so a colleague named Maureen teamed with me to accept work at a time-share resort in Cancun, Mexico. We needed to get to the Denver airport, but neither one of us had a car. I chose an option that is both regrettable and a blessing. I took advantage of Brenda's tenacious grasping for my affection, and I asked to borrow her car.

The only thing I can remember about the day of the accident is the morning at the ranch packing Brenda's car. I know now that I drove, and Maureen was in the passenger seat with Brenda between us.

Was it a horrible mistake or an incredible blessing that we were using Brenda's car? Was it to inflict punishment or to nurture painful growth that God chose to allow black ice to form on our path to Denver?

My feelings of regret over the decision to ask Brenda for the use of her car stem from the fact that I have to admit to using her. My feelings of thankfulness stem from the fact that Brenda was so instrumental in my recovery. Black ice can come in many forms and spin many predicaments into your path.

You think the path is safe; you think it's secure and dry. You begin your journey with the knowledge that others have gone before and done well. So many of the decisions I have made in my life have brought both happiness and grief, relief and discomfort, bliss and despair. If I'm here to learn… I'm learning.

With the advantage of time and the clear perspective that hindsight allows, I now recognize that my greatest catalyst for personal growth and self-discovery was the accident. Of course, I didn't feel this way originally, but now I agree with the philosopher, Nietzsche, who said (and I paraphrase), "What doesn't kill you… you grow from."

I believe that self-discovery is an important, overlooked aspect of the recovery process. If hearing becomes more sensitive when sight is impaired, then is it possible that awareness and the sensibility of the soul are intensified when the body is impaired? The time I spent unable to perform even basic activities forced me to exercise other parts of my being. No, that's incorrect: I wasn't forced; I chose to exercise them. The type of growth that I experienced doesn't lend itself to force or exercise as we tend to think of it. The growth was coaxed by a voice within that could be heard when I was forced to cease the normal activities in my life and allowed to focus on other facets of my being.

I also believe events that happen to us have a purpose. Whatever logic or reasoning was behind the structure and timing of these events, I made progress in areas of my life that I feel are important. There is no indisputable reason for being with Brenda before and during the accident, but I had to deal with circumstances according to my abilities. Significant others may want to consider my experience when assisting, supporting, or prodding survivors through their rehabilitation.

Brenda and I had been admitted to the same hospital in Colorado Springs. While I was lying in a coma, she had been telling my mother that we had made plans together and eventually would marry. I found out years later that friends who knew me in Colorado had been telling my mother that this was not true. In fact, they told her, I was trying to end the relationship.

Brenda and my mother visited me religiously. Shortly before I was discharged, Brenda and I became engaged to be married. What may seem to be a prelude to a fairy tale love story ended after four years. Our marriage created no offspring, and Brenda is happily remarried, 2000 miles away. The first five years following my accident, however, she was instrumental to my recovery. Much of what I have to tell will include her. I could not do this account justice if I excluded her. I would like to stress, though, that this is the factual account of my progress and continuing recovery; it is not the story of a marriage that didn't work.

I realize in my attempt to tell this story, I may raise many questions in the reader's mind about my marriage. As most people who have ever been or are married can tell you, life is complicated and marriage is hard. I was ill equipped to handle my own life, much less marriage. I went through the greatest metamorphosis of my life. I admit I would never be where I am today if Brenda had not been there, but I have to give equal or greater credit to many others. I will never be able to repay her for the irreplaceable role she played, but there are so many in my life that I will never be able to repay. I attempted to repay her the best way I knew how: I set her free. She became free to have the life she is now living.

After I was flown to Peoria, Brenda began to phone me every day at Saint Francis Medical Center. After a few weeks, wearing a neck brace and a cast, she hopped on a bus and came to live with my parents. They took Brenda in because I told them I really wanted her around. She, along with my mother, came to the hospital every day. Brenda moved into my parents' home and, once again,—Yippee, hold on there!—I went sliding on black ice!

Brenda had told me many times that she was not going to spend the rest of her life in South Dakota. I can't accuse her of any intentional, malicious act, but I now feel she unconsciously took advantage of my grasping for attention and affection after the accident. Today, in my mind, I battle between an over-whelming gratitude for Brenda's presence, for the role she played in my recovery, and the hostility I feel toward her for putting me through so much guilt.

Little by little, more people, details and circumstances were entering and complicating my life. Brenda, who had known me for only a few months, made a major decision in her life that directly affected mine. Like a child, I clung to the attention, affection, and security Brenda offered. I'm sure that, following her heart, she acted out of no conscious malice and with no intention to manipulate. However, she had thrown, unintention-ally, major challenges, opportunities, and crossroads into my life. At the same time, however, unlike driving or walking or doing almost anything else, this situation was a part of regular living that I felt I could manage independently. After all, I was twenty-three years old, so whom I wanted to be with was something that no one else had any say in. My life was getting so much more

complex and involved; that's the way life gets as you get older…
and I was aging months every minute.

Like a teenager who grasps for any amount of control he can,
I realized enough about what was going on to know intuitively
that no one could stop me, or wanted to stop me, from being
with Brenda. Why should they have? Brenda was a nice, pretty
girl who clearly wanted to be with me. My parents were in
totally uncharted territory with the whole ordeal. They were just
glad to have me alive. Why would they be resistant to anything
that I wanted right now?

My poor mother didn't know what to think. She had been
hearing different things from different people. Some were saying,
"He was trying to break up with her." And yet Brenda and even I
were saying the opposite. So many confusing, conflicting state-
ments, and all while her son was fighting for his life. She wanted
so desperately to do the right thing. Most people can empathize
with the relief and thankfulness my parents must have felt. Why
would they have denied me any desire that they could have
fulfilled which wasn't obviously harmful? All they really had to
go on was what I was communicating. They had no idea how
immature, clouded, and sometimes tormented my thoughts
were.

Thank God they didn't! Thank God they couldn't know how
chaotic I felt inside. Even when I made the announcement of my
engagement, they only supported me, and were happy with my
decision. Besides, after living with Brenda for a couple of
months, they grew to like and eventually to love her. To this day,
they still send letters back and forth. I cannot say that I regret
marrying Brenda. So much was gained by everyone.

Unfortunately, Brenda and I were not compatible, and I
hope that, someday, our old friends will come to accept that.
There is an important lesson here for caregivers that I want to
stress: my parents didn't try to control me. Looking back now, I

know that, had they controlled the situation, much of what I gained would have been lost.

My recovery was not instantaneous. If it had been, I never would have learned some of the important lessons I cherish. The most important lesson to me? Don't put God in a box! Why do we sometimes feel things have to happen a certain way to be good?

Shouldn't caregivers, both professionals and family members, summon the courage to try not to control all the events that happen? It takes real courage, and real commitment, to take a non-controlling approach to rehabilitation. By concentrating on the survivor's exploration of his or her capabilities, the caregiver can avoid setting specific goals, thus freeing the survivor to gain the courage and optimism to work toward results within his or her own vision. That vision may be as extremely limited as mine was when Brenda and I married.

Furthermore, had I not been allowed to experience the move, marriage, jobs, strangers, and so on, my potential for physical, mental, and spiritual growth would have been aborted.

Frustash... Frustrashion... Frustration!

I could sum up my entire therapeutic experience in one word, and that word is "frustration." Unless you've experienced physical or mental loss and have gone through rehabilitation, you will have trouble understanding the humiliation and the frustration of relearning some activity that you may have, at one time, performed without thinking. After the first few weeks of rehabilitation, I had already regained most of my memory and much of my cognitive awareness. I knew I should be able to do certain things. Not being able to do them made me feel so defeated. People always ask me what it was like to relearn doing this or that. Here is a very simple explanation: it was frustrating! Perhaps through a few examples you will sense that frustration.

Have you ever been asked to do something you've done countless times in the past, but you can't quite remember exactly how it's done? Even a simple task like remembering how to tie a certain knot you tied many times in Boy Scouts, or remembering someone's phone number you've dialed at least a thousand times, but at that moment you cannot recall. Have you ever tried to perform some physical feat of prowess that you accomplished when you were younger, but you're just not as coordinated or as quick as you were at one time? Envision a sixteen-year-old fence climber, who in his eighties can no longer accomplish the task. Try to imagine the feelings of loss and helplessness. During the first several years following the accident, I had feelings like these ninety percent of the time.

I'll never forget the day during physical therapy when my therapist said to me, "Today, we're going to work on going up and down stairs." I wasn't too concerned, because even though I was having trouble just walking down the hallway with someone always hanging on to me, I felt there was no reason I couldn't lope up and down stairs.

The therapist took me to the head of the stairwell, told me to grab the handrail and slowly go down. Thank goodness she clung tightly to the gate belt around my waist, because when I stepped out, my brain no longer seemed connected to my legs! Stumbling over, I started a headlong plunge that I know would have hurt! Tightening her grip, my therapist just pulled me back saying, "Whoa there, not so fast!"

Why in the world did that happen? Why don't my legs listen to me! God… I can't do anything right anymore! I've done this a million times. Maybe if I just do it without thinking about it… it'll work.

I was sure my legs had developed a mind of their own. Just trying to move without thinking seemed to help, but not much. Almost any movement seemed to be a difficult procedure. Some procedures I just forgot, but most processes came back to me almost instantaneously after I was offered a little assistance. Tieing my shoes, for example.

When I started to use my right arm again, one of the things I wanted to do was tie my own shoes. I remember the first time.

As I sat in my wheelchair, I struggled, but finally got my shoes on my feet. Then I held the laces and sat there staring at them.

I know how to tie my shoes! I just can't quite remember how to get started.

My mother, ever present, provided the simple directions I needed, then I clumsily but quickly tied them.

It was strange and it's hard to explain, but there is no rhyme or reason to what things I could remember or what things I had forgotten. Occasionally, I could not remember simple procedures, and at other times, there were complex processes that I had no trouble with, like the procedure to do some mechanical work on a car. The brain is a complex organ not to be easily, if ever, understood. The most frustrating times I can remember having were in occupational therapy. I recall one session in particular.

It was simple enough. All that I had to do was to place these little washers over the ends of wires that were sticking up from a board, let go and they would slide down. I remember thinking as the therapist set the spiny apparatus down on the table in front of me:

This looks easy... cake-walk... I should be good at this because I'm a mechanic. I'm used to handling washers and sliding them on things I can't even see!

It wasn't easy at all. She instructed me to use my right hand to perform the task, but I couldn't even hold the washers by their edges with my right hand. I would concentrate hard on holding the washer by the edges, but my fingers were so unsteady I couldn't do it without the washer snapping flat between them. After I could finally coordinate holding the washer, next came the nearly impossible task of raising my arm six inches over my head to reach the end of the wire.

During the time my right side was paralyzed, my muscles had atrophied so badly that my right arm was like a stick and my shoulder was extremely weak. So, lifting that little washer, to what felt like several feet above my head, was an enormous task. As I would slowly raise my hand upward toward the end of the wire, my arm would start waving wildly back and forth because of my weakness and lack of muscle control. I was so embarrassed; I felt so dumb. I must have looked like a first grade student with a weak bladder trying to get the teacher's attention during class! By the end of the session, I succeeded in getting one or two washers where they should go.

The rest of my therapy during my hospital stay was speech. I basically knew what I wanted to say, but it was so darn hard to say it! I liked speech therapy. The therapist was cute and she laughed at my stupid jokes. Most of the time we would just talk about different topics. I think this therapy was intended to reconnect my thoughts with my mouth. Even if it wasn't the reason, that's what it helped me to do. For several years after the accident, I could not say anything spontaneously. I had to think every sentence through in my head before I could make it come out my mouth. I'll never forget the freedom I experienced years later when I could finally start to speak whole sentences without stopping to think them through.

Imagine the irony. After years of being told to think before I speak, I was imprisoned by the inability to do otherwise.

Although we spent most of our time in speech therapy just conversing, I wasn't going to get through a session without doing some little exercise, which frustrated and embarrassed me. All I had to do was make the sounds *pu ti ka, pu ti ka, pu ti ka* three times over and over again as fast and as clearly as I could. No sweat, right?… Wrong! My mouth was no longer connected to my brain either! As hard as I would concentrate, my mouth would not form the way I intended it. When I spoke, it always felt like I was trying to talk with a big hunk of cheese in my mouth!

Brain injured people with a speech impediment predominantly speak with a nasal quality, which many times, makes people assume they're mentally handicapped. Sometimes, as in my case, they speak very slurred, and people may assume they're drunk. My mouth could not keep up with my mind. My mind wasn't fast, but my mouth and the ability to speak clearly were even slower. Being accused of drunkenness became a familiar experience. I don't blame people who made this assumption, however, because for years after the accident I walked unsteadily and slurred my words. I appeared as though I had had too much to drink. I learned the hard way that appearances can be deceiving.

These are just a few of the accounts I can remember of how extremely frustrating and embarrassing inpatient rehabilitation was for me, but it was nothing compared to the humility I suffered in the years to come. I had some rough moments in the hospital, but consider: those were in the secure, understanding, controlled environment of the hospital, where you're expected to act abnormal or sick. People there are understanding and patient. On the "outside," for years, I felt as if life was a test of how much humiliation and misunderstanding I could take. A few of the people that I came into contact with over the first ten years of my recovery were wonderful, but most people did not have the time or patience to try to understand or deal with someone who did not meet *normal* standards.

So many times I thought I had reached the end of my rope. I became so frustrated, I wished that I had not survived. Sometimes, telling people that I felt this way would make them angry. Especially if the person I told had known someone who had died in an accident or some other tragic way. They felt I was being terribly ungrateful. Thinking back, I realize that this was an ungrateful, selfish attitude, but however wrong this attitude was, I *still* felt this way.

I would like to be able to write: about having an incredible attitude about having nothing but one victory after another;

about possessing an unshakable self-confidence, an undaunted self-reliance, an unquenchable faith in God; or about having and being whatever it is, that makes someone a hero, or someone to admire. But then I would not be writing about my recovery, I would be writing fiction.

I cannot count the times that I felt like giving up trying to improve. I had so many waves of grief come over me, when I wondered why I had struggled so hard and why I hadn't reconciled myself to just being happy with the progress I had made. After all, I got the support I needed; for months, I received Social Security, and Brenda was, more than a little bit, willing to tend to me. I remember thinking—

Why didn't I just quit while I was ahead? Why did I try so hard to impress that doctor? [I was thinking about the annual examination that I had been given to maintain my social security benefits.] *Why didn't I just realize how good I had it?*

Webster's dictionary defines frustrate: 1. to cause to have no effect. 2. to prevent from achieving a goal or gratifying a desire.

Yes, I was **Frustrated**!

Other Happy Events of Hospital Life

While I was in the routine of being awakened at six, wheeled down to the showers, and then eating my breakfast before going to therapy, it became painful to take deep breaths. For a number of days I didn't complain or may have mentioned it only in passing because I was trying to be the model patient. I tried not to complain and only said things I thought people wanted to hear: *Oh yes, that will be fine! or I know, I'm so lucky! or I'm feeling better all the time!* Finally the pain became bad enough that I said something about it to one of my nurses. She called my family physician who came in that evening. He checked me out, listening to my lungs, and sent me to have a chest x-ray. When he didn't see anything on the chest x-ray, he told me to tell him if it got any worse.

After the doctor left I thought—*Well, I'm just going to ignore this and maybe it will go away.* The next day while I was in physical therapy, it became a problem not to be ignored.

It was a simple exercise. All I had to do was get on my hands and knees in the middle of a mat and slowly raise one knee, then the other. All of a sudden everything turned gray and I could not breath!

Jeese, I can't believe how hard it is to do this. Steady... just go slow... concentrate. I'm getting the hang of it! Oh man... what's happening... my chest... man... I can't hardly breath!

[I slid down on my stomach and rolled on my back, gasping for breath]

Oh God... they're going to think I'm a wimp! Let me just catch my breath and I'll get back to it. Man, oh man... this really hurts!

Have you ever had the wind knocked out of you? Well, this was much worse. There I was, sprawled out on the mat, sucking wind like a sprinter. The therapists were frantic. This person rushed in and that person rushed out while my world was steadily turning a darker shade of gray. I finally caught my breath and heard my therapist tell me that help was on the way. My world stopped spinning and I remember wanting to get back to my exercises to make everyone happy, but the therapist told me just to take it easy. My tenacity may have been impressive, but her priority was to calm me down, soothe my anxiety, and pacify me until the nursing staff could come to take me away for some tests.

I remember being rushed on a bed to a testing room and hearing, "My God, his lungs are full of blood clots." All I knew was that it hurt and I was scared. My original injuries may have been much more severe and life threatening, but I had slept through that. This was the first and only time I felt pain and was aware of the fact that I might die. I was rushed to Intensive Care, hooked up to IVs, and plugged into heart monitors.

By this time I could no longer lie flat and breathe without great pain. I was scared. In my extremely child-like mind, I thought—*God why now? I've been a good patient! Why now, after all this?* The look in my mother's eyes scared me even more. Had God spared me in that crash just so I could really see my death coming? I cried.

Needless to say, I didn't die. The blood thinners did their job. After a week or so, I was returned to my big room and my temporary family of nurses and therapists. I undertook the daily routine of being shuffled around to my various therapies, with visits in the evenings by friends and family.

Many of my old friends from church came to see me from time to time. While it was great to see and talk with them, I felt very uncomfortable when they would gather around my bed to pray for me. At one time I had been very active in my church, but I had chosen to move to Florida after coming to grips with an emptiness I was feeling inside. I had visited Daytona several times during spring breaks, and the glitz of the boardwalk and the glamour of the beach scene offered experiences I longed for. Abruptly ceasing all my religious activities, I had followed a passion to live in Florida.

Was the collision in Colorado the action of a punitive God angry at my transgressions? Was it the action of a loving Father offering me a second chance? Or was my decision to move to Florida my first encounter with black ice?

I am grateful to my friends for their prayers, concern, and willingness to give, but I think significant others should be aware of the survivor's vulnerability during the recuperation process, which may seem like an opportunity to impress upon the survivor his need to repent and obey.

Every brain damaged person who has slipped on his own black ice, whether driven off a cliff, struck by a mugger, or exposed to chemicals, each one of us gains a sense of the miraculous. Each one of us feels singled out for survival in order to carry out a special purpose. These feelings are not limited to survivors. They are the feelings of the significant others as well, many of whom have undergone a conversion because the person they love has been spared. These feelings may very well be justified, but that's not the point.

The severely brain damaged survivor's thoughts are too confused to articulate. His powers of communication and logic may be so limited that he cannot debate anyone. Yet, if not pressed with other people's ideas, he may be on the brink of self-discovery. He is mentally immature, illogical, an easy victim to manipulate with feelings of guilt. He needs time, space, and understanding listeners. Not pressure to conform to a particular set of beliefs.

Was I the Prodigal Son? Did God intervene to bring me home to be forever reverent and obedient? Should this be the account of a "wonder boy" or some lengthy parable out of the continuing New Testament? Or is this the real story of a real person with real shortcomings, real problems, an attitude, and with feelings not unlike hundreds of others?

Over the next couple of months I had improved to the point that I became restless. Seeing all the illness around me became unpleasant. My nurses said it was the first sign that I was getting to the point that I should go home. Unfortunately, and quite predictably, Dr. Szymke was not convinced that I was ready. He thought I was cocky and took too many risks. He was concerned about my balance. He felt that two people should be hanging on to me at all times whenever I practiced walking. Although he was, as always, skeptical, he granted me a pass to go home with my family for an afternoon.

It was a chilly but sunny Sunday afternoon in February. My family and Brenda came to pick me up and take me home. I was so excited! I assume I felt somewhat like a prisoner being released from confinement. Everything seemed fresh and new. Throughout the thirty-minute ride to my parents home, I sat there like an excited puppy who was having his first ride in a car. I soaked in the sights as if it was the first time I had seen them.

When we arrived at my parent's home, one of the first things I wanted to do was put on some jeans and a shirt. It seemed like all I had ever worn were sweats and hospital gowns. The house was filled with the familiar smells and sounds of my mother's cooking in the kitchen. I sat in a living room chair taking it all in. God, I felt good! My Mom, Dad, Dan, Lynette, Phil, and Brenda were all there. The scene reminded me of many past Thanksgiving dinners or birthday parties.

Finally my mother announced dinner was ready and everyone started for the table. As Phil started across the dining room to help me, I abruptly grabbed the arms of the chair and unsteadily stood up. I remember someone saying, "The doctor said you weren't suppose to walk around without somebody holding on to you." Dr. Szymke had given my parents strict orders I wasn't to stand or walk alone, but I was on a freedom high and about to overdose. I replied that I would be fine. I was just going to walk to the table, ten feet away. Dr. Szymke was only half-right. I wasn't just cocky; I was cocky and stubborn. Head-injury victims tend to be that way.

As I made my way slowly toward the table, everyone stood and watched me with wide-eyed anticipation. "Easy now," someone said. I walked across the carpeted floor with smirking confidence, stepped off the carpet onto the hardwood floor of the dining room and *Whoosh!* In my stocking feet, I slid downward, slamming my head against the hollow-core door of the stairway and *BAM*! As I lay there, you could hear a pin drop. For a long second, everyone had frozen in shock. No one moved except for Phil who had already made it over to me and was bent down to help me up. As he helped me to my feet, I started laughing uncontrollably! I thought—*This is so great!* I had been under the blanket of tight protection in the guarded hospital environment for months. I couldn't go to the bathroom without someone hanging on to me. Someone always was touching me! Someone scrutinizing every move I made!

This tumble felt fantastic! I had fallen down and I didn't shatter into a million pieces!

When I consider the past ten years, this was the first time since the accident that I was allowed to act independently and literally fall flat on my face. I know that allowing me to try different things had to have been scary for my parents, but I was so stubborn, that letting me try and letting me fail was their best and only approach. As it turned out, throughout the course of my recovery, failure was never quite as bad as expected.

As Phil helped me to the table, everyone assured me they failed to see the humor in this and I had better not pull that stunt again. Everybody calmed down. We spent the rest of the afternoon eating and joking around. Evening began to fall and reality set in. It was time for me to return to the hospital. Oh, I didn't want to go back, but spring was coming and it was time for new beginnings. I knew that I would be coming home soon.

Dr. Szymke came in late the evening of the next day to check on me and see how my furlough had been. Being the cocky kid I was, I couldn't resist the temptation to tell him of my little incident. Quite expectedly, he scolded me, abruptly telling me to stand up and walk toward him. Sure that I had things under control, I walked across the floor to him. He watched as he nodded his head approvingly and said, "Not bad, not bad." I thought—*Well, there's a first time for everything.* Then he said, "OK, now walk a straight line."

Yes, I'm ready for this! You humiliated me with this before, but I've been practicing!

I had told my therapist about him asking me to do this trick once and we practiced a little everyday. With a sarcastic grin, I walked a straight line, heel to toe, like an alcoholic practicing for his next binge. He said, "Not bad. Now walk it backwards!" I froze. This was unexpected. As I moved slowly backwards, my brain once again seemed to detach all circuitry to my legs. I started to fall over and Dr. Szymke reached out, held me firmly, and said gently and kindly, "See, you're not as good as you think you are." (He was an old softy at heart after all!) Not only could I not speak spontaneously, it was hard to perform even the simplest physical feat without rehearsal. My body simply did not seem to remember how to do many things.

To some degree I was glad I had to start over from scratch on most things. I was in physical therapy one day, practicing walking up and down the hall with my therapist alongside. I was having trouble with balance, so my therapist was having me try different things to better control myself. I told her all my life I had walked pigeon toed and was very self-conscious about it. She exclaimed, "Oh, OK!" as if we had stumbled across some treasure. She told me to walk pigeon toed if I felt more comfortable that way. I refused, saying that if I had to learn to walk all over again, this time I was going to do it right. Maybe it took me a little longer than it would have to get the hang of it, but it worked! I no longer walk pigeon toed! I had gotten a second chance at life. I was determined to overcome any shortcomings I was aware of. I wanted to learn things right this time.

Mind Games

What is *normal*? What is Dave Fierce's maximum potential? What is *normal* for Dave Fierce? A brain injured patient's biggest obstacle to mental recovery is in the patient's own perception of himself. Remember when dealing with your brain injured loved one, he or she sees himself or herself as being *normal*. Probably the most difficult part of my entire rehabilitative process has been the mental recovery. This has been very hard because it is almost totally subjective. There are so many unanswerable questions.

During the last week of my hospitalization, a clinical psychologist came in to administer my IQ test. I remember that she split the test up and only tested me for a short while each day, to accommodate my attention span. Although there were puzzles I could not put together and pictures I could not understand the meaning of, I felt I had done an adequate job and scored average. I was to find out months later that I had scored in the mentally handicapped range! I was shocked! I thought, yes, I had some rough spots, but that test was hard! My mind would justify my shortcomings without my even trying.

One of the first, most noticeable things about my mental state was my over-reaction to every little emotion. If anything were even remotely funny I would laugh much too hard and much too long, like Horshack on "Welcome Back Cotter." If anything were sad I would start to cry like Stan of "Laurel and Hardy." I was aware that I was over-reacting, but I could not control it. This emotional lack of control was most noticeable whenever I would try to tell a joke. As I would get to the punch line, I would speak louder and louder; then I would start to laugh so hard I couldn't speak clearly. All my life I've loved comedy and being comical, but, at this stage of my recovery, I hacked up jokes so badly that anyone laughing could only be laughing at me. One of the first signs that my mental capacities were returning to me was found in my abilities to tell jokes and to see a humorous slant in a situation.

Another characteristic indicative of my mental state was the fact I could not seem to keep my mouth shut about anything. Whatever came to mind, no matter how embarrassing it was to others, or myself, no matter how tactless or hurtful it was, it came out. In the same way a child will walk up to someone and ask, "Why are you so fat?" or say, "My Mommy says you talk too much;" I would blurt things out, oblivious to possible repercussions. While this behavior may be understood and tolerated coming from a child, I am afraid my commentary hurt and alienated many people dear to me.

After I had been out of the hospital for about a month, I was one of the first survivors to be enrolled in a cognitive therapy program sponsored by Easter Seals, designed to help rehabilitate the brain injured. The program was like school in the respect that it lasted six to eight hours a day, Monday through Friday. The therapeutic activities centered on independent living skills. We prepared food, took a bus to the grocery store to learn how to get around without driving and how to handle money, laundered clothing, and performed many other basic, daily functions. One activity that sticks out in my mind was relearning how to write checks.

We all sat down around a table. The therapist gave us pens and put mock checks in front of us. Like so many times recently, I was unable to get started when she instructed us to fill the check out for one-hundred dollars. I sat there and stared at the paper.

I know how to write out a check! This is so easy! Why can't I remember how to fill in the written number part?

As the therapist talked us through the process, memories of writing checks popped into my mind. I remember justifying my hesitation to myself by thinking—*Well, it's just been so long since I've written a check.*

We also used flash cards to relearn our multiplication tables. Memorizing my "times tables," as we called them in grade school, came quickly to me and it only took a few repetitions for me to memorize them all, but at first I could not recall them. I remember justifying this to myself by thinking—*This is no surprise because I use a calculator all of the time.* Again, my mind performed instant justification. The aspects of this therapy centered on thinking processes and mental health.

The program arranged for each of the participants to meet individually with a psychologist once a week. One week the psychologist did something that put me into depression for the first time since the accident. She interviewed us individually asking us casual things about ourselves while she used a camcorder to tape the session. The following week without any preparation, constructive commentary, or helpful remarks, she played it back for us. As I watched I thought—*Oh my god, do I really act and sound that way? Jeese… I'm a nerd!* I remember I went home that day and asked my mother and Brenda if they would tell me about all the characteristics of mine that were weird or different. I became obsessed with the fact that I could not trust my perception of myself anymore.

My mind was flooded with confusion and doubt as I tried to remember all my recent interactions. I tried to remember if I had done anything stupid or embarrassing. As I worked to remember, I came to the realization that my perception of these memories could not be trusted. The results of using video to point out the abnormal characteristics I exhibited were devastating. Was I supposed to be shamed into acting *normal*? Was the end result of this humiliation supposed to be that I would never act socially inappropriate again? The message I heard was: See what you do! Act *normally*! Unfortunately, seeing myself act *abnormally* on TV didn't change the way my brain worked. If whatever processes my brain used to judge my behavior hadn't improved, then I would still be doing the same inappropriate things. The fact that I knew I was acting inappropriately didn't help me improve, it only made me feel like a geek.

The brain-damaged survivor is in an unique category of mental deficiency. Those with brain damage have the potential for growth. Unlike the person with a birth defect or brain degenerative disease, I was somehow able to improve all of my cognitive abilities. If brain cells don't regenerate, then I trained some of the extras I had lying around. If the procedure of video-taping had been done along with preparation and follow-up, this technique may have actually have been constructive, but done as it was, the whole thing just served to degrade me and made me feel inadequate. I may not be educated in psychology or well versed on modern therapeutic practices, but the abruptness of this approach left me stunned. Please don't slap your survivor in the face with his or her shortcomings.

I became fascinated with a person's self-image and how an individual's defense mechanism could project them into a fantasy world if necessary. A person's self-image is crucial to the ability to handle life. I've spent some time talking with a young adult who had Down's syndrome. When I asked him if he felt bad because he had Down's syndrome, he replied "no" and said he felt perfectly *normal*. He didn't think of himself as different and disliked it when people treated him that way. This is exactly how I felt. Think about it: do you feel bad because you can't perform brain surgery or understand quantum theory? No, of course not (unless you're a brain surgeon or a physicist). We all tend to gravitate toward a feeling of satisfaction with our own abilities, as well we should. People need a healthy self-image to manage and cope with the continual onslaught of life's setbacks.

For about eight years after the accident, my mental capacities increased at a phenomenal rate. I was relearning my twenty-three years of development, starting from square one, both physically and mentally. As I gradually improved physically, my mental limitations became more and more of a stumbling block. I started moving and speaking better so people's perception of me and expectations of my abilities were increasingly incorrect. I was embarrassed about my limitations so I would do things to make people treat me *normally*. I would let them do most or all the talking. I would move around as little as possible and use my left arm only. I succeeded in having people treat me *normally*, but I failed to communicate the fact that I had limitations. I was tremendously self-conscious about not being up to speed with the rest of the world. But because of the strange paradox of self-perception that I experienced, even if I had realized that I was not up to speed, I would have thought, "that was in the past and now I'm better." I never had a clear picture of who I was.

At any given point during my recovery, except recently, I've been able to look back and reflect upon my reactions to a particular situation which occurred only a year or two before and realize my emotional reactions were abnormal or completely disproportionate to the circumstance. I would think back to a certain event and remember how I was thinking, how I was feeling, or how I saw things. I would realize it was exactly how I thought, felt, or saw things when I was around fifteen or sixteen or some other age in my life. My profound error was, at any point during my development, I always felt like I had attained mental maturity. I always thought—*Wow, I'd never act **that** way or say **that** again. Now I'm **normal**.* It was always a secure feeling. I would feel like I had been there before; it worked out then, so it would work out this time. Now nothing is familiar; as I reflect upon situations that took place during the past several years, I realize that the way I have thought and reacted is unlike any prior experience. Now, I'm no longer repeating stages of development that I already experienced in my teens. I'm breaking new ground. I finally have caught up with myself.

For roughly six years after the accident, I felt like I was living in a dream state. Of course, I didn't realize this until I started to come out of it. You very rarely realize you've been dreaming until you wake up. For six years I was in Dave Fierce's skin, living Dave Fierce's life, but life was a knee-jerk reaction. Most of my commentary on different topics was what I had heard others say or what I thought others wanted to hear. I really didn't speak with my own voice. I repeated things. Since it was so hard to speak spontaneously, I spoke what was already in my head instead of originating new thoughts. This mental state of cloudiness and people's perceptions of me were some of the hardest, if not the hardest obstacles to overcome.

The mental capacities of even a slightly brain injured survivor can be affected. I have known people who have only been knocked unconscious for a short time, and some who have only suffered a concussion. Both report memory deficiencies or increased agitation. Although the mental side effects of brain damage are ill defined and subjective, significant others need to be aware of these things and remain constantly conscious of the problem.

I realize the difficulty that a significant other faces when trying to give latitude for their survivor's mental struggles. They battle with the argument between the survivor having true and honest deficit, or simply using their injury as an excuse. There is no litmus test for the validity of mental shortcomings. There are no black and white standards or a set of guidelines to follow. This can be most troubling. There really is no comprehensive answer. Significant others need to constantly keep the potential for a problem in mind and deal with every situation as it arises. One should always keep in mind that we live in a world with others who have as much right to be here as we do. We should, no matter what our mental state is, be held accountable for our actions.

Take your loved one's mental state into consideration and realize that even though their deficient mental state may be the reason for their actions, it does not excuse them from responsibility. Everyone, no matter what their state of mind, needs to take responsibility for their actions. Even the friend of mine who has Down's syndrome is held accountable for his actions. No matter what reason a person has for being at one level or another, no one has the right to abuse another.

Try to help your loved one to understand and accept their individual limitations. Be as objective as you can and then approach the survivor with honesty and respect when conveying any assessment to them. Remember that the survivor views himself as *normal*.

I don't have any set of "golden rules" that I think you need or should follow in coping with or preparing for the survivor's mental handicaps. I only know that my thinking processes and mental state were immeasurably altered. Dealing with these changes are confusing and distressing for both survivor and significant other. Patience and love need to be exercised by the significant other and a sense of personal responsibility needs to be instilled in the survivor. Convey to your survivor that they have a right to be as simple minded or clever as they want to be, but manipulation or being hurtful is never acceptable. Although the survivor needs to be accountable for his actions, remember that their perspective of their actions may be skewed. They will see themselves as thinking and behaving normally. Be careful when assessing your survivor's emotional reactions, viewpoints, or behaviors. Remember that just because they act or respond differently than they did before, it does not make it wrong. Make your assessments more from the standpoint of healthy or unhealthy, and less by right or wrong. Above all things, continually remind your survivor of the progress they have made. Support and praise should be the tools used most. In almost every case, better results come from praise for a positive behavior than from accenting a negative.

Coping with the mental deficits I had was the most demoralizing thing for me. The biggest problem was, I never realized that I was making a mistake at the time that it happened. Realization would always come much too late for me to redeem myself. I still recall my past actions and occasionally want to crawl into a hole because I'm so embarrassed that I behaved or responded a certain way. Please utilize all your patience, respect and sensitivity with your survivor when dealing with something as subjective as their mental state. The one golden rule that I do have is for both survivor and significant other… the "Golden Rule." Treat each other the way you would like to be treated.

Life on the "Outside"

I was released from the hospital and felt a mixture of excitement and apprehension. I was moving back in with my parents in their little country home and the whole affair had the haunting feeling of permanency about it. Had people been right? Was I returning to live with Mom and Dad, to be taken care of the rest of my life? *Not if I had anything to do with it!* My parents had taken great pains in preparing the house for me to live there. My father had installed hand-railings on all the stairwells, put a hand-held shower in the downstairs bathroom and set a kitchen chair in the bathtub, because I could not take a shower while standing up yet. My mother had prepared the guest bedroom for me, so I wouldn't have to climb the stairs to my bedroom. Perfect, Brenda slept upstairs in my bedroom and I slept downstairs across the hall from Mom and Dad. Because I couldn't climb stairs alone, this was a livable arrangement for my Mennonite mother and father. They also would be close to me in case anything should happen. What more could happen, right? Life, that's all. "Life is something that happens to you when you least expect it." Didn't Ben Franklin say that? Right!

I do recall one more life threatening incident happening a few days after I was out of the hospital. I guess living in the sterile environment of the hospital had lowered my resistance to germs. I'm not exactly sure what happened, but I became ill with an extremely high fever. I do not remember all the exact details probably because my fever was so high that I was delirious. The only incident that really sticks out in my mind now is that Lynette had come to the house, frantically stripped me naked, and plunged me into a bathtub of cool water. This entire incident is hazy. I'm not sure of all the detail. I am not even sure of what was wrong with me. Whatever it was, it passed and I remember feeling angry. I don't even know who I was angry at, but I was so sick and tired of being sick. All this drama was wearing on me.

I began a new routine. Feeling sorry for me, because I had to deal with my strict hospital routine of waking up at 6:00AM, my mother let me sleep until 7:00AM now. Every morning she would get me up and put me in the shower, I would eat my breakfast, and then we would go down into the basement to practice walking and skipping. Because of my paralysis, my right arm would tend to curl into a fetal-like position whenever I concentrated on walking. At the same time, my right leg had atrophied badly, and was extremely weak. It would try to curl up, and refused to extend fully. The outcome of this unconscious tendency of my right side was to make me appear like the Hunch-Back of Notre Dame, minus the hump, shuffling across the bell tower. Mom would hang on to my gate belt, and we would lope back and forth across the basement floor. Try as I might, I could not get my right arm to stay down along my side while I concentrated on walking. It seemed that I had to chose: I could have my right arm hang at my side naturally, or I could walk. I didn't like this option, so I would stick my right hand in the back pocket of my jeans as I walked. This forced my arm to stay down at my side. Mom and I would lumber through this for about an hour and then it would be time to drive into Peoria for out-patient therapy.

At the outpatient clinic, Dr. Szymke assessed me periodically and I had all the usual: physical, occupational, and speech therapy. Different therapists—same humiliation. I remember on one occasion, Dr. Szymke was assessing my progress by having me close my eyes, reach out to my sides, and try to bring my arms in to touch my nose. I touched my forehead, my mouth, but I'd be "danged" if I could hit my nose! I felt like a complete basket case, but I wasn't going to give in. No matter what my therapists wanted me to do, no matter how embarrassing, I gave it my best shot. I would spend several hours at the clinic and go home.

At home I would sit around with Brenda, watch TV and plan our wedding. (She planned, I agreed.) Sometimes friends would call and Brenda would drive me to their homes. In the evening, I would eat my dinner and watch more TV. Many nights, after the 10 o'clock news, I would shuffle out to the sidewalk or the road in front of my parents' house. There, in the secure, cool darkness of a country night, I would practice trying to jog, skip, and jump rope. I also honed my skills at taking a fall! My brother, Dan, came home from college on the weekends and his presence was extremely comforting and helpful.

The first weekend I was out of the hospital, Dan decided that I needed a night out. He took Brenda and me to a movie! I was so excited! Although Brenda and I spent all of our time together, and Dan was going as a "third wheel," it felt like being a freshman in high school and going on a double date with your older sibling! I felt every emotion one experiences while preparing for a first date. I remember getting ready to leave and I was filled with anticipation. I got dressed up for the first time in months. I felt so embarrassed about having to put the gate belt on around my waist, but wearing the gate belt and letting Dan hold on to me when I walked was a prerequisite for this "night on the town."

I don't remember all the details of the trip to the movies, but I remember sitting in the theater being so excited that I could hardly sit still. An event that sticks out in my mind happened when we were leaving the theater. We waited until the room had all but cleared. I got to my feet, walked up the aisle, and Dan helped me cross the lobby to the exit. As Dan held the door with one hand and firmly held my gate belt with the other, a young man who was obviously in a hurry came rushing in the exit. While my mind said that the thing to do was to just move aside and let him pass, the connection from my brain to my legs had not yet fully linked and the sudden change of direction sent me toppling down toward the floor. It was a good thing Dan had a tight grip and easily held me in an upright position. Dan gently held me with one of his arms and stuck his other in the middle of the guy's chest. He just said, "Hold on there buddy! You want to just take it easy!" The guy just stood there wide-eyed and open-mouthed. He stared at me and stammered, "Oh… sorry." Dan helped me across the parking lot and into the car. I felt so secure! As I have said many times since, the younger brother had become the older! After all the abuse and teasing I had given him over the years, he wasted no time in assisting me with my needs. He may not even remember this incident, but my love and respect for him deepened that night. I admire him greatly.

Among the more humiliating times I had adjusting to this new life, was one evening when Brenda and I decided to go to a small town fair. One episode that sticks out in my memory is when I was just walking through the crowd trying not to get pushed over. I was walking in front of some children and I overheard one of the little girls say, "Look at that man. He's really drunk!" I stopped dead in my tracks, as they walked by giggling and staring. I've been told over and over by well meaning friends that I just shouldn't let things of that nature bother me. I should just let them roll off my back. How many times have you been told similar things and you know they're right, but they still bother you? Then Brenda and I decided we wanted more excitement out of this experience than corn dogs, French fries, and root beer floats. We saw the ride called the "Octopus" and thought, "Why not?"

That decision was a big mistake, but I guess I needed to find out just how bad my equilibrium was. I clumsily climbed into our little pod on one of the arms of the "Octopus" and, eyeing me warily, the attendant pulled up the bar designed to hold you in. I knew that I was in trouble when, while still just rotating around slowly to let the rest of the passengers in, I already felt the corn dog in my stomach protesting. The machine started slowly and steadily built up speed. About the second time around, I realized I had made a terrible mistake. Every time we would scream around, hitting our apogee, I released some more of my greasy, barely palatable, dinner. It splattered against the street below and people went scattering. Poor Brenda, she was yelling at the top of her voice at the attendant to, "Stop!" She only succeeded in drawing his attention to my predicament and I'd bet he thought I was just drunk. I'm not sure, but I think he saw me and pulled back on the lever to speed up the ride. The Sea-Creature-From-Hell finally slowed and the attendant made sure we were the last couple off. He smirked as Brenda helped me down the stairs of the platform. As I passed by him we locked gazes and I thought cynically and sarcastically—Carneys! What a breed! Ya godda love 'em! Brenda helped me over to the grass of the park and I must have lain there for half an hour. No drunken experience I ever had felt that bad.

Several weeks after I was out of the Hospital, Brenda and I decided to drive to Florida for a couple of weeks. My parents freaked out; they couldn't believe we were going. Although their fears may have been warranted, everything went OK. Brenda did all of the driving, of course, and I did all the resting. It was so good for me to get away from everything and for the first time I felt independent. Naturally, Brenda took care of everything and I was away from the reminders of the accident, surrounded by sights and people who reminded me of my life at the height of my independence. Although I dearly loved my family, I was out from under their suffocating, watchful eye. I'm sure they tried their best not to be over-protective, but this was all new to them and they weren't sure what the boundaries were. After all, I was twenty-three years old. They weren't terribly over-protective or they would have refused to let me go. But here I was; havin' a blast, soakin' in the sun, messing around with my friends and trying to mess around with Brenda!

It was a horny teenager's dream comes true! Two weeks with my fiancée, nothing to do, nowhere to go, and sleeping in the same bed! It was our first night in Daytona and my dreams became just that, nothing more than the activity of my brain. My brain was the only thing ready to go, no other part of me seemed ready. I was on substantial doses of Phenobarbital for seizures and to this day I assume that's what caused my problem. I couldn't get an erection. Sometimes I could, but then the duration was uncertain at best. My dreams had turned into my worst nightmare! I thought God had played the worst kind of practical joke ever.

Anything but this!... Not this!... Take my legs!... They're not much good anyway!

This is an embarassing topic to discuss, but one that I think needs to be addressed. Taking into consideration the fact that two thirds of those who sustain head-injuries are under the age of thirty-four, sex becomes a significant subject. I know that for most young head injured survivors sexual frustration can be overwhelming, causing them to do incredibly self-abusive or harmful acts. Be conscious of these drives when dealing with your survivor.

I dealt with one young male survivor whose biggest dilemma was sex. He was a junior in high-school when his accident happened. He had been a good-looking football star and a very popular student. He had no trouble getting dates to the prom, so to speak. Although his physical features hadn't been changed, after his accident he moved slowly and in an uncoordinated manner. He spoke with a nasal quality. Needless to say, his attractiveness to the opposite sex was significantly reduced, and he was no longer as successfull with dating as he previously had been. He could not bear being undesirable to the women he was attracted to. Having the same emotional instability that I had in the early stages of recovery, he was driven to incredibly self-destructive behavior. If I have helped even one survivor or caregiver by bringing this subject up, then it has been worth the embarassment.

When approaching the topic of sex, much sensitivity, caution, and sometimes counseling have to be exercised with your survivor. This is especially true if your survivor was successful with dating relationships in their previous life before their injury. The realization that they are not perceived in the same way as they were in the past is an earth-shaking revelation to survivors. Usually, especially in the beginning, survivors do not realize that they are acting differently and cannot understand why people are acting the way they are towards them. Even though physical maturity governs their hormones, emotionally they may be extremely child-like.

Having Brenda in my life was important in many ways, but as I reflect, not having to deal with the girlfriend factor was probably one of my biggest advantages. Brenda's presence and willingness provided the companionship that most head injured survivors need. I didn't have the obstacle of loneliness and isolation to overcome. Sexual drives are so powerful. If the drive goes unsatisfied, it can lead to overwhelming depression and can cloud all other thinking processes.

In spite of all the aforementioned difficulties, we had a great time and came back to Illinois. I continued my daily routine of doing my own tailor-made exercises at home and going to the outpatient clinic. As driving is a mark of independence, I became obsessed with getting behind the wheel of a car again. I continually bugged my mother to let me drive. She would take me to parking lots, just like when I was fifteen years old, and let me take the controls. Sometimes my mother or Brenda would just let me drive along the country roads. I remember going down a back road once when, unexpectedly, two or three cars went by from the other way. Suddenly, I felt confused. This was the first time there was anything going on around me that I had to be aware of. I got over to the right so far that I almost clipped a mailbox. I laughed it off, acting as if it was something I was trying to do in order to scare Brenda. As soon as I progressed enough, they started letting me drive to town with them. I always felt like I was drunk, just for an instant, when cars around me were passing or turning. I knew that I dare not say anything about these episodes because I wanted to drive! Every time I saw Dr. Szymke I would ask if he felt I was ready to drive again. Even if I saw him pass by in the clinic, I would stop and bug him about it. He finally said he would have me retake the IQ test to see where I was.

The same psychologist he sent to the hospital returned to administer the test to me again. She knew I had been bugging Dr. Szymke to give me permission to drive again, so she was a little skeptical as she gave me the test. She would set the puzzles in front of me, and I would speedily put each one together. As she showed me the drawings, I had to laugh. Why hadn't I understood these before? If I hadn't remembered some of the images in front of me, I would have sworn that this was an easier test. The psychologist was impressed! I had made a considerable jump in my score. She said I should go to take the driving test and try to get my license reinstated.

Significant others should be cautious about letting a loved one drive again too soon. Yes, loosing the privilege of driving a car does feel devastating to a person. Survivors I've spoken to have told me about their frustration with this. Yet, however badly I wanted to drive again, looking back, I was not ready.

Significant others need to look for signs of the survivor becoming panicky or confused while driving. Don't become a back seat driver or let your own nervousness rub off; just be aware of what's going on. I remember shortly after I had started to drive again, I became confused and ended up driving the wrong way down a one way street. In spite of my inner short-coming, which I was able to conceal, I started driving again and thankfully without incident. With the ability to drive again and my progress in outpatient therapy, I felt a new sense of independence. I had progressed to the point where my therapists at the clinic felt there was little more they could do for me.

I remember the feeling I had the day I went to the clinic and my physical therapist told me I had come to a place she could do relatively little more to help me. I was ecstatic! I had set a one-year time limit for myself. I had determined that I was going to be just like I was before—in one year. Here it was, less than six months after my accident, and my therapists had cut me loose! I knew my judgment of my abilities might be cloudy, but here were unbiased clinical professionals, saying I had improved to the point they could do no more! I was ready to face the world. I was ready to marry, get a job, and resume a *normal* life! After all, if my therapists thought I was good enough, I didn't need to worry about other people's impressions any longer. If I was considered able in the eyes of a scrutinizing professional, surely I was fully prepared to face the world! I had no understanding that while they simply meant I was ready for independent living, that "being like I was before" was not only an impossibility, it was not their intention. So when my mother approached me about enrolling in a cognitive rehabilitation program, put on by Easter

Seals, I only agreed because I thought it would be fun. I even had vain imaginings of the people at Easter Seals coming to me during the first few days and telling me I was much too advanced to be in the program. I'm glad, now, that I didn't realize how far I had to go or how long of a journey I was embarking on, because I would have become terribly depressed. My biggest obstacle to overcome was my self-image, but it also has turned out to be my salvation. I'm now glad I never saw myself in a true light. If I had, it would have had the effect on me that a child experiences when they're constantly reminded of their failures. I would have been thrown into a deep depression and consumed by self-pity, thinking, "I'm so far off the mark, why should I even try?"

On Your Marks... Get Set... CRAWL!

I have already spoken a little about my cognitive rehabilitation provided by Easter Seals. We not only did the things I've already mentioned, we also had many computer software programs that we used to work on our spatial recognition, long and short term memory, vocabulary, reflexes and coordination, and other thinking processes. I especially remember the work I did with a computer program designed to help improve short-term memory. It involved memorizing an ever-increasing series of one digit numbers. I became so proficient at memorizing the sequences that I was soon challenging everyone, including the therapist.

A problem with memory is the one side effect of brain damage that can be generalized among survivors. I have never spoken to a survivor who didn't have problems with short term memory, long term memory, or both. However, I am living proof that memory, like any skill, can be improved.

As a significant other who must, at one time or another, rely upon the memory of a survivor, hearing—"I'm sorry, I forgot," can be very frustrating. If this happens several times, the excuse of the survivor's being brain injured can wear very thin. Please exercise patience and compassion, but recognize that your survivor has to take some responsibility. The degree of responsibility will depend on his or her level of recovery. Survivors have to realize that many people without any type of injury have problems with memory.

There are many memory aids available, as well as memory building techniques or simple processes which can be followed, such as mnemonic procedures or making lists.

It was my last couple of weeks in the cognitive rehabilitation program, the end of August, with a beautiful fall approaching. I turned twenty-four and I was going to be wed to a beautiful, somewhat impatient, but caring young lady. Brenda and I frequently argued, but I accepted the clashes as results of wedding jitters or my own mental obscurities or the fact that she was always right. Maybe it was a mixture of all of these, compounded with a few more things. I didn't know and my mind was so cloudy. I was living in a dream and this was where the Dream-Maker was taking me. I went along for the ride.

I think back now to how I saw the surrounding circumstances of my wedding and I realize that this is exactly how I felt about life and viewed things when I was around 15 or 16 years old. I had neither concern for nor expectations of the future. I didn't think about the fact that I was making a decision that would affect the rest of my life. What was the "rest of my life" anyway? This was fun! Some of my old college buddies, ones that I hadn't seen in years, were coming to participate in the wedding. Planning the trip to South Dakota for the wedding was like planning a road trip when I was in college! The best part about this party was that I was going to be the star attraction! I was the center of all the attention. Everyone followed my lead. This was my party and my friends and I were organizing a blowout! I was in control again. I planned my own destiny. I had spent ten months being told when to sit, when to walk, when to eat, how to eat, how to walk, and how to feel! I should feel *lucky*; I should be *grateful*. I felt like a human pet! No more! I called the shots. It's my party and I'll act like a mental midget if I want to!

A week before the wedding, Brenda returned to South Dakota to start setting things up. I felt even more independent. I had a whole week to spend in total freedom. Now I could drive and Brenda wasn't with me twenty-four hours a day. Although I was getting married in a week, I felt like I was on the loose, and I didn't think about what I was doing.

Brenda knew exactly what she was doing. She had suffered much, but her injuries did not effect her judgment. I, on the other hand, could not see past the end of my nose. The whole affair was a big party to me. I had no realization of the long-term effects of what I was doing. I lived only for the moment. I pray that someday Brenda can forgive me for any injustice I have done. However, what's done is done. Brenda and I were married in Canby, Minnesota and had a big reception twenty miles away in Gary, South Dakota. For my family and friends who couldn't make the trip, we had another fairly big reception at my parent's home in Illinois a week later. During the following week, a local news channel decided that they wanted to produce a human-interest story about my recovery.

The story mainly centered on the rehabilitation I received in the Easter Seals program. I recorded the news spot on video tape and I watch it occasionally. As I watch it now, I remember what I was thinking and feeling while the news reporter interviewed me. Strange as it seems at this time, I remember feeling that I was at the end of a long road and about to embark on a totally new beginning. I even told the reporter—*I feel the wedding is a culmination of all that I have been through the last months.* I actually believed that because I had been through a three-month hospitalization, undergone outpatient therapy, participated in the Easter Seal program, learned to drive again, and gotten married, that it was all over! I thought I had been through my rehabilitation period and it was over! I sincerely believed I would move back to Florida and never have to be bothered by this accident again. I had no idea of what was in store, of just how far I had yet to go. I didn't realize my process of learning and growing had just begun. A week later, towing a U-Haul loaded down with wedding presents, Brenda and I set off to live in Florida again.

We arrived in Daytona Beach and I felt so exhilarated! As Brenda and I had said over and over again, we were moving back to Florida and were going to get on with our lives. Our lives had been consumed with nothing but the accident for over ten months. I remember feeling many times that I would never live another day without thinking about the accident. Every morning, the first thing that popped into my head as my feet hit the floor, was the accident. I would reach for something and have to use my left arm and I would think about the accident. I would brush my teeth or comb my hair or walk downstairs or try to communicate a point I had to make, and I would be reminded of the accident! The accident, the accident, the accident! As hard as I would try, everything I did, every situation I got into, would remind me that I was not the person I used to be. Here I was, trying to launch a new life for myself, and I felt that I would spend the rest of my days tormented by **the accident**!

While trying to settle in and start all over, a Daytona Beach police officer pulled me over for a minor traffic violation. After he asked me a few questions, he was sure he had pulled over a drunk and asked me to step out of the car.

Oh boy! This should be good. If I get a DUI Brenda will kill me!

I cautiously opened the door and stepped out of the car. I tried so hard to appear *normal*. I know now that if I got a DUI there is no way they could have made it stick, but I didn't think of that then. Here I was, with no alcohol in my system, about to be judged by how well I could walk a straight line or touch my fingers to my nose! Thankfully, I had been pulled over by a compassionate officer who listened to my pleadings and excuses. He gave me a test where I followed his light pen with my eyes. He asked me where I lived, and told me to drive straight home.

When I lived in Daytona Beach before, I had just completed a real-estate course, but had never taken the state exam. After Brenda and I were in Florida for a few weeks, I applied to take the test. Brenda had gotten a job as a receptionist at a time-share resort and I had already spoken to the sales manager about working there as a salesperson. I had sold time-share properties in Florida before, and that's what I was doing in Colorado. Although time-share resorts frequently hire unlicensed individuals to be salespeople, after the interview I'm sure the sales-manager thought I was somewhat slow or slightly retarded. He told me I should take the exam and that if I passed, he would talk to me further about working. While the Florida real-estate exam has a reputation of being one of the toughest real-estate exams in the nation, I attended two review sessions and passed the test with two or three points to spare! During the time between taking the exam and finding out the results, I got my first job since I tried to slide off a mountain.

I came home after the informal interview and felt so proud. Brenda would be so happy! It was the tourist season in Daytona Beach, so I had little trouble getting a job as a "go-fer " in a souvenir shop. I remember that when I told Brenda, her response was less than encouraging. Brenda and I still argued frequently and I never, oh but never, was right. Despite whatever was upsetting Brenda, I started stumbling around the gift shop five or six evenings a week trying to appear *normal*. I did really tough things like stack seashells and open boxes of Daytona souvenir key chains. I think back to some of the interaction I had with the other employees and realize that they must have thought I was a little slow. The night manager of the store just thought I was goofy and after a couple weeks I received a phone call from the owner telling me that my services were no longer needed. It didn't hit me too hard because on the same day that he called, I received my real estate test results in the mail. Now I could go out and get a real job, "selling time" at the resort where Brenda worked.

I talked to the sales manager the next day. He was surprised when he found out that I had passed, and while he seemed a little hesitant, he set me up for training. I think that he and the other management people at the resort thought that I would never sell anything. While I don't think they would have hired me under normal circumstances, Brenda and a good friend of mine worked there, and I know they felt obligated. Because I was licensed, I was paid on commission. If I never sold anything, they would never have to pay me and I would quit. I think management felt safe in their decision. My first week went by and I talked to many clients, but I didn't sell anything. I felt terrible because when I had sold timeshares before, I was some-what of a hotshot salesman and had done well enough to be offered a job as an assistant sales manager in Colorado. But all our doubts and bad feelings soon appeared to be unfounded; at the beginning of my second week I sold a timeshare condo-minium!

One of the sales managers told me afterwards that he was amazed. He hadn't expected me to sell anything. Over the next few weeks I became more comfortable and started to sell at an average pace. Asking me if I was drunk or high became a familiar question I received from clients, so I incorporated a little expla-nation of my accident into my sales pitch. I timed it carefully so that when we had talked to the point where I was sure that they were wondering about my manner, I'd explain—*I was involved in a head on car collision and spent four weeks in a coma. So no, I'm not drunk. Among the many things that I can't do well yet, are walking and talking.* I sold timeshares for about a year and during this time, physically and mentally, I kept getting better. Slowly, ever so slowly, but surely, I just kept getting better and better.

As a salesperson, my greatest tool was my mouth. To speak clearly, I had to silently rehearse every sentence in my mind before I could say it. I constantly had to remind myself to speak slowly. Speaking slowly just supported people's assumption that I was drunk or slow. Because I could not speak spontaneously, I had a fully written-out, memorized sales pitch. I even had canned jokes prepared so that I could be humorous at the right time. (Most of them were lame!) So while continuing to undergo my own home-brewed therapy, including exercises like trying to run and skip, I came up with my own therapeutic training to help my speech. I had tremendous difficulty reading aloud. The pathways connecting the eyes to the brain and then the brain to the mouth had become rusty and they would no longer run smoothly. So I would go to my room to be alone and I would practice reading a book aloud slowly. At first, when I say slowly, I mean very, very slowly. Sometimes I would time my pace and force myself to hold every consonant and vowel sound for two to three seconds. I felt like I was re-training my mouth to form each sound. Little by little I would pick up the pace, but the first time I would slur a word, I would slow it way down again. It worked, and in much less time than I expected! I would encourage anyone who has trouble speaking to do this. There were so many tough and humiliating times.

One of the toughest obstacles I faced was one that I didn't even realize I was faced with, until years later. On the surface, I no longer appeared to be very bad off. If you would have asked one of my friends in Daytona about me, they would have said something like, "Well, Dave has a little trouble walking and talking and sometimes he's a little uncoordinated and slow, but otherwise he's *normal*." They had no comprehension of the internal struggles I had to deal with at the time. The main problem was that they didn't care. My biggest obstacle to overcome was the fact that I was surrounded by people who were not close to me and couldn't comprehend what I had already gone through. I tried to explain to people, but I was so tired of explaining myself to everyone! I'm sure that people felt I was exaggerating or trying to excuse my indolence. I started noticing a certain *look* that I always got.

I became an expert at recognizing the *look* on people's faces. (Sort of a pre-occupied, wondering *look* that they always got when they realized something was wrong with me.) I would meet someone, talk to him or her awhile, maybe do something, and they would get that *look*. They had noticed some little movement or a slur in my speech, and they realized that something was wrong. I would see that we had passed the point of no return.

I had progressed far enough to be capable of independent living, but not anywhere near to the point that I was capable of meeting other people's expectations of me. In many ways this was good for me. I was around so many people I had just met, or had known since I had returned to Florida, and their expectations of me drove me to continue trying to improve. If I had stayed around my family and friends, my development would have tapered off. They were so impressed by my progress and they knew that I had already exceeded what was expected of me. I would have attained and remained in a condition that had been others' prognosis for me time and time again. I would have reached a "plateau." So many friends told me, "Don't *worry* about what people think!" But dammit, that's so hard to do when you've spent your whole lifetime being treated and perceived a totally different way.

Although being around a totally new crowd, a crowd of people who judged me and reacted to the person I was at that time, I did not escape the frustration that every survivor of serious brain injury faces: the rejection by friends. During spring break one year while living in Florida, several of my friends from college came to Daytona. We got together a couple times during the first few days they were in town. Toward the end of their vacation, they noticeably started to avoid all contact with me.

I drove out to the hotel they were staying at. Cornering one of them, I bluntly asked about their avoiding me and he said—"I don't know, Fierce… you just changed, man. I mean… I don't know… you seem like you've recovered okay from the wreck and everything… but you're just different." I felt like he had pulled my stomach through a small hole. My mind was reeling.

What?!… nothing happened… I didn't do anything… Why? What did I do?

I asked him as much, and he just said, "I don't know, man! Just that… some of the shit that yer doing just isn't cool."

I was blown away. I just wanted to explain and I went into a lengthy dissertation on what I thought would change everything. He just nodded his head and said, "Okay… okay… okay, buddy. I understand… it's just that some of the other guys don't understand what's up. It's okay."

I've seen him once since then.

This is a devastation that so many survivors of brain injury must confront. Significant others should prepare for this. There is not any way that I can think of to avoid this. A survivor is changed. There are not any rules to the types of change, but you can be assured of it. My very few close friends remained friends; they just got used to the new me, but my casual, "partying buddies" fell by the wayside. The people close to me cared enough for me to put up with my eccentric behaviors.

One friend in particular told me something that I will never forget. It had been a while since I had seen this person and he was remarking on how much progress I had made in the two years since he had seen me.

We were just sitting in his pick-up truck, parked in front of my house, with the doors open, listening to the radio, drinking a coke on a warm summer afternoon. We talked about what we were doing at the time, what had happened since we had seen each other, and he was commenting at how amazing my recovery had been. Slowly and sheepishly he said, "Ya know Fierce... I have to admit something. Right after your accident... I didn't really like to hang around ya. It was sorta like... like... havin' a retarded younger brother around." He then looked at me side-ways, hoping I wasn't going to be upset with his honest, blunt commentary. I paused at first, then I broke into a laugh and thanked him for his honesty. I realized that he had just explained so much about the reactions of so many people!

A survivor many times will gain a different set of priorities, and will have to make new friends. A survivor will be changed, but change is not always for the worst.

Recovering from brain damage is like recovering from alcoholism in the respect that there is no stopping point. If we're here to learn, everything that happens to us helps our learning, and we will never reach a stopping point. When someone asks me how long will it take to recover, I ask them how long they expect to live. Recovery is a process, a process without end. We only get better at working with life; we never conquer life. Why would we want to?

I've reached the point in my recovery where I appear *normal*. Would it benefit me to feel I could finally give up? Of course it wouldn't!

This is the cutting two-edged sword of my philosophy of life: a person needs to find his place in life and be content with it, but never give in to limitations. When I say to be content with your place in life, I'm talking about finding your own pace or rhythm. Without an acceptance of yourself as you are right now, you are only sentencing yourself to condemnation and hopelessness. There are so many survivors out there who become overwhelmed by others' perceptions of who they are today. After being treated a certain way for the years prior to their accident or illness, they can't accept their image today.

The person your survivor was no longer exists. Like a butterfly from a cocoon, let the new person emerge. Encourage your survivor not to become depressed and indulge in self-pity. I didn't like the way people treated me, but it only motivated me to dig in and try harder. I had plenty of my own pity-parties, believe me, but when I got down, that's when I'd force myself to remember my friends' advice about not worrying about what others thought. My friends were right. Don't *worry* about it, *do* something about it! The balance between striving to overcome and struggling to accept yourself is critical. When I talk about accepting yourself, I am not talking about complacency. I may have traveled light-years from where I began, but I haven't arrived. Now, I just may be physically and mentally equal to the masses, but it's the fool who gives up trying to improve himself.

Toward the end of the two years Brenda and I lived in Florida, I started selling appliances. One evening during this time Brenda and I were invited to a dinner party given by some friends. After dinner we sat in their living room just to talk and let the meal digest. Someone was talking about an Eskimo and his thin wife. I was listening to this and suddenly I said—*Yeah, you show me an Eskimo with a thin wife, and I'll show you an Eskimo with a heat pump!* Everyone just roared! It wasn't the fact that the joke was so funny, it was the fact it came from me! I remember that my friend's wife just sat and looked at me in disbelief. I was shocked too. I couldn't believe it popped into my mind, and even more unbelievable was the fact it came right out! I didn't have to silently rehearse the gag before I said it! It came out fairly slurred, but it happened. For me, this marked the beginning of my head starting to clear. I was aware it was happening, and I was also suddenly aware that I had been walking around in a daze. I didn't know why this was happening or exactly how this was going to affect me, but everything started to seem so much clearer. Over the next few weeks, thoughts started to pop into my head, and with just a little conscious effort to keep my speech slow, I could say what I was thinking. This was terrific! I didn't experience this all the time, however. At first, I only felt this sort of clarity of mind perhaps once a week. As time went by, I had the experience of feeling "clear minded" more frequently.

An important change was in what I saw when I looked in the mirror. I noticed that when I would get ready in the morning and look at myself in the mirror, I saw someone looking back... ME! As my mind started to clear, there was a certain blank expression, a vacancy in my eyes, that had started to go away. It's hard to pin down exactly in words, but other people said that they noticed it also. I felt more alert, more aware of what was going on around me. It was like I had been dreaming for three years and I was slowly awakening.

As your survivor starts becoming more aware of what's going on around them and increasingly becomes "clear minded," it can be an exciting, sometimes troublesome, almost scary thing to watch. Brenda was excited by any progress I made, yet it created more friction between us. She was trying to get accustomed to me, and I just kept changing. Whether she consciously realized it or not, she was losing control over me. I'm not saying that she wanted to control me. I use the expression, "losing control," in the sense that she was losing any sense of security that she had gained from knowing how I was going to react. Your survivor is going to continually change and grow, if you let them. They may reach a point that you feel they are "out of control." As this change begins to become more dramatic, it may become unsettling, and sometimes unhealthy. Extreme sensitivity has to be employed to let the survivor experiment with new thoughts and feelings, while trying to keep them within the boundaries of self-preservation and common courtesy. Don't make the mistake of trying to keep them "under control" and end up anchoring them to a "plateau;" you may be responsible for indirectly or unconsciously halting their development in your attempt to keep them in a familiar spot.

Twenty-six Year-Old High School Student

While working sixty hours each week at the appliance store, I started thinking about returning to Peoria to go back to school. I brought the subject up to Brenda and she was adamantly opposed. I just let the topic die at first, but it just kept coming up in conversations and I felt strongly that I should. I knew that I had come a long way in my physical recovery and I felt that returning to school was exactly what I needed in order to recover mentally. It was July and I knew I must make some decision soon or wait the school year out. I decided to approach Brenda once more with the idea. She was just as opposed this time as the first. However, as I had started to become "clear minded," my thinking processes had started to become more logical and when I had a point to make, I could now make it.

For the first two years of our marriage, if Brenda and I disagreed, I could not express myself and I would always yield to her wishes, even when I knew I was right. Whenever a disagreement would arise, the harder I would try to express myself, the cloudier my mind would become and the more slurred my speech would get. The outcome was that she made most of the decisions. Without getting into the details, let me say that we arrived at a decision to return to Peoria where I would enroll in a local junior college. I gave my two weeks notice at the appliance store and the manager was shocked. He said, "You spent weeks bugging us and hanging around until we finally hired you, and now you're going to quit?!" He was right. With my slow, slurred speech and obvious physical limitations, they really didn't want to hire me. But they needed sales people and being paid on commission, I'm sure that they felt like the management at the time-share resort. Regardless, two weeks later I was off on another new beginning.

Brenda and I loaded up a U-Haul truck and towed our car back to Peoria once again. We arrived a few weeks before the fall semester began. We took the time to find an apartment, got settled, and I visited some of my old therapists to tell them what I was up to. They were amazed at my progress in the last two years and were excited about my decision to return to school. When I told them that I had decided to go into physical therapy, the reactions I got were discouraging. None of my therapists actually came out and said that this goal was beyond me, but they all cautioned me about the rigorous academic requirements and tried to persuade me to go into something easier. This was just another challenge to me. Like my attitude toward Dr. Szymke, I thought—*They say I can't? I'll show them who can't!*

In August of 1987 at Illinois Central College, starting with some remedial high-school level course-work, I began my college career with an obsession to prove that I was just as capable as anyone else. I studied long into the night and in-between classes. What I lacked in raw intelligence, I made up for with sheer tenacity and finished my first year with straight A's. I started to actually have, not only days, but weeks go by during which I didn't think about the accident. Although I still walked and talked a little strangely, most people didn't seem to notice and I felt the nightmare of the accident fading. When I graduated from ICC, it had taken me three years to get to a level most people arrive at in two, but I finished with a 3.8 grade point average on a 4.0 scale.

During my last year at ICC, Brenda and I argued constantly. It became painfully obvious that we had different priorities in life. I realize that I have an opportunity that most do not: a chance to document my side of the story. I realize that I have the opportunity to set the record straight (my version of course) and to get the final word. But I'm going to resist the temptation to do so and remain focused on the purpose of this work.

Casting blame is pointless and futile. In the end, no one wins and all are hurt. I will admit that I have made so many wrong decisions; I made so many wrong moves. I am the last person that has any right to judge anybody. But finally, after years of pain and loads of guilt, I made up my mind that I was not going spend the rest of my life paying for a decision that I had made in an immature state of mind. I chose to do what I honestly thought, then and now, was the best for everyone: I asked for a divorce. I also made a decision to pursue a career in health information management and was accepted into a program at the University of Illinois at Chicago.

The two years that I was in the Health Information Management program and living on campus at UIC were two of the roughest years of my life. After all the events of the last ten years, I honestly see these two as exceptionally tough.

The campus at UIC is located near the southwest of Chicago, not the best part of town. I lived across the street from the infamous Cook County Hospital, where most of the victims of gang-related violence are taken. I lived in a small three-bedroom efficiency with two roommates that I had never met before and who could barely speak any English. They were good-natured guys, but between their class load and my own, I seldom saw them. Out the window of my cramped room, ten stories up, all I could see were buildings and more buildings. No horizon, no sunsets, hardly a tree. At night and during school breaks, everything on campus was closed and locked tight. I needed a key with an ID to go anywhere or do anything. There were security guards and fences everywhere. I soon learned that you just didn't go out at night. Living within the inner city, surrounded by four different hospitals, I longed for the rare moments when I wouldn't hear a siren wailing or a car alarm blaring. I found a part-time job working second shift as a medical record clerk at a hospital in the south of Chicago. For a boy who had been raised in the country and enjoyed living on the side of a mountain, all this intensely urban life was almost too much to bear.

Did I also suffer because Brenda was no longer in my life? Let's contemplate this idea.

If I maintain that coming out of a coma and progressing through the stages of my rehabilitation were, for me, equivalent to birth and maturing through childhood, then I would have to say that Brenda had been with me all my life. My second life anyway.

This leads me to the conclusion that, yes, even though I never would have admitted this to anyone and was fond of saying – *Never look back*, yes, I suffered.

Brenda was a part of my life. And in the same way that prisoners go mad for the lack of their tormentor's abuse in solitary confinement, I was totally alone, longing for the companionship of even someone who seemed to dislike everything about me. Meeting and overcoming challenges without Brenda being there, if only to point out the grievous error of my ways, was an almost insurmountable challenge in itself.

I am so glad that now I have found peace in my life, and have risen above the guilt, pettiness, and shallow attacks. I am so glad that all my strong, painful emotions over this whole ordeal have been stomped out and I am only left with a hot, smoldering, deeply embedded bitterness. A bitterness I can now define.

Is this more therapy?

Before I had moved to Chicago I had a long conversation with one of my friends, and I came to a decision. I decided to not tell anyone I met about my accident and, in most every case, I held firm to that decision. During the two years I lived in Chicago the subject rarely needed to be addressed. I made up my mind to not use my accident as an excuse. The few times I did mention it, I just gave a rough outline of the events.

Speaking somewhat slurred and having many days I was extremely tired from late nights of study or work, I must have sounded and walked like I had come to class drunk or high. I thought I was doing reasonably well and was successful at appearing completely normal, until the end of the first quarter, when some of my classmates were shocked to see me at the "Breakfast with the Dean," and had no qualms about telling me so. "Breakfast with the Dean" was a continental breakfast held at the end of every quarter, attended by administration, faculty and students on the honor roll. Fellow classmates who also made the honor roll were constantly coming up to me that morning telling me they "just couldn't believe I had made the Dean's List." When I asked them why, they just told me "they didn't know why, they were just surprised." A few days later, I asked one of the students in the program about the other students' reactions. He told me he had heard other people in the program talking and the scoop was … "Dave's kind of slow." I was floored! I felt that I was never going to get beyond others' superficial, judgmental, baseless, impressions of me!

One day I was being critiqued on my progress in the program by one of my teachers; she was being very nice and helpful to me. She asked many questions about my past and my family life. She kept questioning and probing, asking about my curriculum at ICC and why I had waited until so late in life to go to college. It seemed to be a strange line of questioning considering that there were people in my program older than I. She seemed rather uncomfortable and was obviously digging for something. When I told her I used to live in Florida and I liked the pace of the south as opposed to Chicago, she exclaimed - "Oh, OK! That explains why you seem so laid back!" I believe that she used the phrase, "laid back," in place of "slow." I was irritated and resentful! My living situation was hell for me. I was working very hard in a tough program, working from sixteen to thirty hours each week at my job, going through some significant personal problems, and trying to deal with condescending people who consistently estimated my abilities based solely on standards of quick, precise, and graceful speech and movement!

I would like to tell significant others this type of snap judgement is one of the most devastating, emotionally traumatic, humiliating, and frustrating obstacles that I seemed to come up against constantly. Most of the survivors I've talked to express the same frustration. This particular type of response from people is a frustration that is so powerful, that I find it very difficult to depict in words. I really have no definitive answers or a canned approach to handling it. Maybe the answer lies in the individual. It is not a generality. We have to accept the reality of the situation. This snap judgement is the kind of response that is not going to change. The best I could do was deal with the ignorance on a case by case basis.

I look back on the last ten years of my life and think—*What did I expect? Can I blame any of those people who judged me so callously, so insensitively?* Have I not done the same or something similar? So, who's wrong? Is it that 98.8% of the population is wrong and should be held accountable for the error of their way? Probably... but it's never going to happen, and thinking and obsessing about it will only frustrate, depress, and anger you. If the brooding goes on too long, you only end up buying an Uzi machine gun and spraying the local grocery store. People aren't going to change. The masses are not going to suddenly become compassionate, patient, and understanding. I don't have all the answers, especially for the question of how to overcome this particular frustration. However, it may be helpful just to be sensitive to this when dealing with your loved one. Maybe all the pains can't be eliminated, but that's OK. Emotional pains never kill, and if we continually refresh our perspective on our circumstances, we can grow from them. This is how I dealt with the frustration of being misunderstood again.

The result of confronting these adversities was to make me reassess my progress. I thought—*I feel so much better!* I knew I walked and talked better, but these cold, insensitive reactions to me made me start to re-think and doubt my progress. Working as a traveling nurse, my sister had contracted to work at a Chicago hospital. Lynette only lived a few miles from where I was, and her presence gave me the strength I needed.

Lynette and I spent many evenings together just talking and watching movies. During one conversation, we began to discuss my progress and some of the reactions I was receiving from people. When she told me she noticed certain things, certain inconsistencies, picked up little movements, and dysphasia in speech, I felt at first that she had slapped me in the face! I thought—*No... I'm not like that... oh sure, when I'm tired maybe you can notice little things... but I'm OK... I'm OK* (what I failed to recognize before talking with Lynette... I was OK)! I will say it again, I am so thankful for my family's support! Lynette just listened to my fears and feelings of inadequacy, reassured me over and over, but had enough love and respect for me to give me an honest, straight forward evaluation.

The way she reassured me was also very helpful. She didn't coddle me and say, "There, there, Davie. People just don't understand how much you've been through. You're OK. Don't listen to them." She just had more of a clinician's attitude and stated very matter-of-factly, "It's no big deal! People are going to do that. You just have to be thankful for all you've accomplished and go on with it." She always said everything with concern and caring in her voice, but she never said the little "nice" or pseudo-loving things people say to smooth a situation over. Lynette practiced "tough love." She was always ready to give help, but she was never willing to act for you in lieu of your acting on your own. She always let me know I was OK, doing great, and had accomplished so much, but she didn't patronize me.

Although she showed a somewhat cold, objective attitude when summarizing my progress, she never once alluded to the fact that I should or could do more. I never felt she held anything but respect, amazement and thankfulness at my recovery. Although I felt no pressure from her to accomplish more or improve beyond any point, her response made me dig in again, and try harder.

I started to become self-conscience all over again. I started reading aloud in my room again, slowing my speech, and speaking as clearly as I could. I was conscious of every movement I made. I slowed everything down again: my speech, my responses, and my movements. I stopped saying anything in class. Before, I was always stating my opinion, always volunteering to be the spokesman for group projects, always volunteering to be one of the first people to give a report to the class, but no more… no more. I hung back. I didn't volunteer anything. I tried to be totally inconspicuous. I stopped killing myself to get top grades; I just wanted to get out! It was the last leg of my program and the teachers relentlessly loaded us with homework. If I had not been so close to getting my degree, I fear I might have quit.

It occurred to me that over the past several years, a few of my friends had referred to me as "wild eyed." I stared at my reflection in the mirror for hours, paying close attention to the involuntary movement of the right side of my face. I noticed that when I squinted, only my left eyelid would noticeably contract; that when I smiled, only my left eye would crinkle. I put on a happy face, a sad face, a surprised face, any face; my right eye would stay wide open. This was a result of my right side paralysis.

Before the movement started to return to my right side, I smiled a half grin and spoke out of the left side of my mouth. The right side of my face was like a dead man's. Not only were my right arm and leg paralyzed, but also the whole right side of my face. During the time I was in a coma, my right eye would not close and cream had to be put on my eyeball continually. With the scars on my forehead; the thin, uneven way my right eyebrow had been re-attached; and the tendency of my right eye to remain wide open; I had a bulging, wild-eyed look! I was totally unconscious of the confusing messages my facial expressions were sending. The grimaces on my face did not reflect my state of mind. Thus, making faces at myself in the mirror became a new therapeutic exercise for me! I would smile and make a conscious effort to crinkle up my right eye and raise the right corner of my mouth. I would squint and make an effort to squint both eyes evenly. Even now, my right side still lacks some of the sensitivity and feeling that it originally had. Making sure my face was responding correctly by watching myself in the mirror, I would teach myself what a correct expression felt like. By over-exaggerating my right side facial movement, I taught my face how to move, in the same way I taught my mouth to form different vowel sounds

Survivors, along with significant others, have to be very careful not to confuse effort with accomplishment. There are still many things I cannot do, or can only do without the speed or grace I once had. There are many things I haven't accomplished. I realize that I've mostly written about the things I've accomplished and the struggles I had while trying to achieve them, and chose not to dwell on the many failures and disappointments

I've had. This has been done as more of a service to the reader than anything else; the content of this book would be much too lengthy and boring to include all the shortcomings. It's not the accomplishment anyway! Whether or not successes make for better reading, the important matter is found in the effort! I don't want the reader to think that the "pot of gold at the end of the rainbow" is the object to look and hope for. The "pot" may not be there and nobody can say what it would look like if it were! Rainbows are not painted or looked at for hours because there's a pot of gold at one end. Rainbows are beautiful! Enjoy the rainbow of life! Don't try to avoid the struggle of life. We're here to learn and grow. The effort of growing matters, not the reward.

If you concentrate only on the reward, you'll become impatient and frustrated. You have to remember that rewards come in many shapes and sizes. When you look only for reward, you have a definition of what form it should take. While looking so hard for something specific, you may walk right by something very valuable. By struggling hard to overcome obstacles in Chicago, I gained so very much, but I came close to missing the rewards because they were so different from the ones that I was seeking.

While I was living in Chicago my mother called me and gave me some unnerving, unsettling, saddening news. A young man very dear to me, who I hadn't spoken to since I left Peoria, had a terrible accident. To paint the picture, allow me to regress a little.

The cognitive rehabilitation program I had attended was held in a building directly behind Saint Francis Medical Center. During my lunch hour, I visited with the people I knew in the rehabilitation unit. There I met Dennis, a young man, still in high school, who had been involved in a car accident and was severely brain injured. The nurses and therapists all told me that Dennis reminded them of me and that his progress paralleled mine. When I first met Dennis he was unable to speak, so he just sat and smiled as I spoke to him. I returned to the rehabilitation unit several times over the next few weeks to visit Dennis and to reassure him. Although I gave him advice and encouraged him, he was well on his way to recovery and I felt I was with a kindred spirit. I married and moved to Florida, but when I returned to Peoria and school, I sought him out. His progress was amazing, but I was not surprised.

Over the months to come, Dennis and I became close. We spent many hours together bike riding, playing ball, doing exercises, and discussing the problems he was having adjusting to his new and scary life. We went places together, I introduced him to my friends, and I felt in many ways that I was his mentor. He became an inspiration to others, volunteered his time to patients and families, and took on the responsibility of being a leader in the head injury support group we attended. Now I recognize that Dennis had fallen prey to the same immature attitudes and mental set backs that I had experienced. He said some things that, at the time, were very hurtful and I stopped spending time with him, even though I understood better than anyone just what was going on in his head. I knew his real opponent was time and that he was doing just fine. Dennis was suffering through the same impatience and frustration I had experienced. I was unable to relay some of the lessons I had learned, because I had not yet progressed far enough down the road of recovery.

Dennis, I wish you could have given me and yourself time!

Oh God, I know when tragedy strikes someone you love, the tendency is to blame yourself, but I can't help but feel that if I was geographically closer, we could have talked. While I was far away in Chicago, dealing with my own problems, Dennis became too weary with the struggles of all that had happened and the future he faced… and shot himself.

Oh how I wish he could have waited ten years!

Dennis' mother has become a terrific advocate for the head injured and has written a book herself. Why is there so much pain before things change?

After Thoughts… Ten Years After!

I rarely bring up the topic of my accident anymore. Thank God I no longer need to explain my behaviors. Although I still seem to end up talking about it, I gloss over the details and just try my best to summarize the whole thing. Even people who think they know about it, unless they've known me from the beginning, know relatively little compared to the extent of it. When I do mention it, people will say something like, "Wow, I never would have known." Praise God! That's such a treasured sentence to hear! I have worked so hard to get to the point at which I am no longer hindered by the after-effects of my accident. The biggest reason I choose not to mention it or to gloss over the whole thing is the fact that I find it increasingly difficult to believe that I was, mentally and physically, so far away from where I am today, even though I was there. I'm afraid that if I go into any detail, the person I tell will think I must be exaggerating. Most people don't really care about what you've done. The only thing that matters is what you do. In time-share sales we had a saying—"You're only as good as your *next* sale." Most people are really only concerned with how your actions affect them. That's OK, because ten years after, I continue to improve and to achieve in all areas of my life. The improvements are more subtle now, but thank God I only have subtle improvements left to make. I struggle with life now just like everyone else. Finally, I am no longer struggling just to reach the starting block. No one should be impressed by what I've achieved. Hell, I'm not even impressed anymore. I'm not seeking anyone's admiration.

So ten years later I've rehabilitated to the point were I walk and talk just like a *normal* person. So what! What does that mean? Does that mean everything had a happy ending? No… it's not over. Now I just face different challenges. Things like never making quite enough money, love relationships, job hassles, what kind of car I should drive, do I look fat in these jeans, etc., etc. So I've gotten to *this* point, but it really would be nice to be at *that* point. It will never stop, but is that so bad? Learn to be excited by the progress of your loved one, but just remind them to never give up. Accomplishing this or that is not the point. The continual effort is the point

Your pride and happiness with their progress should be evident, but do not ever give the impression that it's time to level off. Progress, accomplishment, and usefulness are relative; they're a matter of perspective. A weak trait in one situation is almost always a strength in another. Let yourself be excited over your survivor reaching little goals and don't be embarrassed by show-ing excitement. You may feel ridiculous for showing excitement over something you consider simple or useless, but your showing excitement may be exactly what is needed to motivate the person. Never make the loved one feel as if their accomplishment or progress is not important. Take example from my experience. I started out encouraged by the praise I received for opening milk cartons by myself and sought in those close to me the inspiration I needed to continue to the point I am now. Never slap your loved one in the face with his or her shortcomings in an attempt to prod them into action or effort. Don't thoughtlessly remind them of the same things everyone else does.

Finding out who I really am is not just *one* of the important things I've learned. It's the *most* important thing. All the other "important" issues in my personal life seem to be taken care of by my natural response to them as I learn more about myself. I struggle daily with revealing more of myself to me. I find wisdom in the Bible, the Tao Te Ching, The Prophet, and many other writings of people past and present. Knowledge and insight is all around us. Help your loved one on their journey by helping them find out who they are now. They are not the person they used to be, but they can be so much more! Help them to stop trying so hard to reclaim their life and to start enjoying who they are now. Support your survivor. Help them to appreciate their abilities and not be frustrated by their inabilities. An important lesson for me to learn was - be good at what you're good at and don't beat yourself up over what you haven't accomplished.

Furthermore, don't focus or teach your loved one to focus on outcomes. There is one occupation none of us will ever have (in reality): Fortune Teller! We can't predict the future! None of us knows how things will turn out. The best we can do is be ourselves; whatever that may be.

My desire is that this work reaches those whose life has been spun into turmoil by head-injury, stroke, or other debilitating injury. From the family members, who now have a loved one who seems strange and unfamiliar and who are trying to understand and cope with the feelings of guilt or loss while they struggle daily with the burdens of care and financial responsibility, to the survivors, who may have spent a lifetime learning about themselves only to be faced in the mirror by a stranger. Survivor, if you're reading this - It's all right to experience conflict and emotional pain. It's all right when you can't do all the same things in the same way you did. You are a precious individual, a rare treasure. Find these things out for yourself. Stop dwelling on what you could do and concentrate on what you can do now and the effort you make to do more. Don't just throw in the towel and decide it's not worth it.

I have a cartoon summarizing what I want to tell significant others, and survivors of brain injury or any other debilitating injury. It is a drawing of a stork standing in a pond. This stork has scooped up a frog and has the frog's head in its mouth with the body and legs sticking out. Hanging by his head, this little tenacious frog has reached around and has the stork by the throat in a death grip. The caption reads... **"Don't ever give up!"**

I know a girl who was confined to a wheelchair for fifteen years and can now stand up! Some time ago I spoke to her and she told me she was getting married, but not until she could walk down the aisle! I love this attitude! I don't care where you're at in your recovery, or how long it has been, you can still progress. Maybe I was given all the "lucky breaks", all the support from family and friends that I could ever want, but I bear no sole ownership to the rights of progress. I have never seen anyone struggle against the odds of rehabilitation and come away totally bankrupt.

When I first was injured, nearly all I heard about from the doctors and therapists were references to "plateaus," a romantic sounding piece of pseudo-medical jargon I believe may have been designed to ease the consciences of those who grew weary of trying any longer. It may have been a label born of misunderstanding and fear. They all told my family and me that head-injured patients would always progress to some certain, undetermined level of improvement and then "plateau." There are no plateaus! Until disease or the natural aging process takes over, there is never a point you cannot improve! This has been proven over and over in the field of body-building. Muscle magazines are always running stories about little old Mr. Jones, who at the age of 60 has been working out and now feels better and has more dexterity than he had ten years ago.

One thought is so important to me that I'm going to write it in capital letters: THIS ALL TAKES TIME… IT TAKES TIME… IT ALL TAKES TIME!

Significant others and survivors, beware of reading this book and thinking to yourself… "Oh, now I've got it!" Please understand that, having written this book, I haven't got it… how can you have grasped it from these pages? I only offer my own experience, my own reflections, my own… whatever! Every individual case is just that, individual. My thoughts and explanations are only my own. I relate only my viewpoints in the hope that they may help others in similar circumstances, but not by offering any sort of blueprint or roadmap.

I just recently let a survivor of a minor head-injury read my work-in-progress. She was tremendously excited and was talking so fast about it that she would stumble over her own words. By some of the things she was saying, I could tell that she was thinking—"Now I got it!" Who have you read about recently that would probably have said something like that? Could it be me?

It is exactly *that* kind of thinking that continually threatened my progress. Had I not constantly changed my environment, constantly surrounded myself with new people and new jobs, I might have reached the feared plateau!

Very few survivors are in the same situation I was in. Most brain-damaged survivors have lives and responsibilities they need to return to. When my accident happened I was traveling to Denver Airport in order to catch an airplane and start my life over again in Mexico. I was a restless, risk-taking, adventure-seeking time-share sales person. After only a few phone calls, I had set myself up with a job "selling time" at a resort in Mexico.

When I had come to the decision to move from Florida to Colorado I sold my car and was able to pack all my possessions into Brenda's car. I didn't need a car in Colorado because I ate, slept, worked, and played at the ranch. I rarely took the fifty-minute drive down the side of the mountain into Colorado Springs. So when Maureen, my friend from the ranch, and I decided to jet off to Mexico, I took advantage of Brenda and borrowed her car. So at the time of the accident, because of all the support that was given, I had no responsibilities or loose ends to tie. My only responsibility after coming out of the coma was to recover. Twenty-four hours a day, seven days a week, all I had to do was **get better**!

While I climbed the ladder of rehabilitation, I suffered endless embarrassment, but who would laugh at what has now been over a decade of perseverance? One of the most valuable pieces of advice I could give significant others is to tell your survivor to suffer the humiliation of recovery. They shouldn't be afraid to try and extend themselves. If they don't try, they'll never do anything. Yes, people laughed at me behind my back, but "He who laughs last…" My biggest challenge in life is with myself.

I especially feel for survivors of minor brain damage because they may have only been unconscious a short time, only hospitalized a few days, and the people around them may expect them hop right back into doing whatever it was that they were doing before. The survivor may expect the same and will not understand their own reactions or shortcomings. Our brain is the most complex, most poorly understood organ of our body. The types and severity of complications from damage to that organ are indeterminable. If there were a set of known rules to the complications, then there would be set of known time frames for recovery.

This book is not meant to give excuse to the brain injured. It is an attempt to give hope to those affected, and an understanding of a widely misunderstood injury. As I progress further and further, I can relate more and more with the frustrations that you, as a concerned significant other, may feel. I don't have all the answers. I can't look into the heart of anybody and see his or her motivations, but neither can anyone else. I only know that we cannot help being affected by aspects of brain injury that often include memory loss, increased agitation, impatience, social dysfunction, clouded and disorganized thinking, bitterness, resentment, blunt commentary, impulsive actions, and a whole plethora of physical disabilities. Similarly, we cannot avoid all the frustrations that significant others feel.

My suggestion to survivors: don't give up trying to better yourself. Don't give in to laziness and excuses, and don't take the easy way out. Don't give up trying to keep a positive attitude, and don't try to give out false impressions of yourself. Don't *ever* give up!

My suggestion to significant others: listen closely to your survivor. That doesn't mean coddle, pamper, baby, or indulge, but listen and give thoughtful assessments. Take notice of everything, no matter how insignificant it may seem to you. Help the survivor to exercise good judgment without being authoritative. Try not to control everything. Always exercise love and respect. And realize… it all takes time.

The End of the First Mile

Despite the things that happened to me during the two years I lived on UIC's campus, I went on to graduate in June of 1992 with a Bachelor of Science degree in Health Information Management (formally known as Medical Records Management). I started sending out resumes about two months before I graduated from UIC, probably thirty to forty resumes in all, to different parts of the country, mostly to places with warm weather. The first resume I sent out, for practice and as kind of a joke, was to Saint Francis Medical Center (SFMC) in Peoria, Illinois. It was the only resume I sent within the state of Illinois, but I felt like SFMC was my alma mater in a strange way.

I really didn't expect to hear anything at all from SFMC, but about three months later, I received a letter saying that there was an opening as a supervisor in the Health Information Services department, inviting me to come in for an interview. I've been working now as a supervisor at SFMC for almost three years and during the first few months I passed the national exam to earn my credentials as a Registered Record Administrator (RRA). Working at SFMC enables me to take advantage of opportunities to thank some of my caregivers.

Every now and then I will pass a nurse in the hall or help a physician who took care of me as a patient. The emotion I feel is incredible when I see and talk to these people. Shortly after I began working at SFMC, I made a special trip to the rehabilitation unit to visit a nurse who played a particularly important role in my life during my hospital stay. I walked up behind her, just stood and watched her. After a few moments she turned around and looked me in the eye. It may have taken her a few moments to recognize me because my hair was shorter, I had no beard, I was wearing a suit, and I was standing up! She just let out a squeal of happiness, said "Oh my God!" and embraced me tightly.

I continue to try and better myself physically, mentally, and spiritually. I refused to learn to write with my left hand, so I still write slowly and people will comment and make friendly jokes about it sometimes. I still stink at throwing anything, from softballs to Frisbees®, but I still try it every chance I get. I was never any good at the big three sports (football, baseball, and basketball), but I'm one of the first to jump in and play at family reunions or outings to the park with my friends. I try my best no matter how embarrassing it may get. I just try really hard not to make the losing play for my team.

Recently, I tried water-skiing for the first time in my life. The whole scene must have been like watching a Jerry Lewis movie! My reaction time is slow so I bought a weight machine to help improve my considerable right side weakness. My right side is still weaker than my left, but at the age of thirty-three I'm in better overall condition than I've ever been. That makes me feel even better about myself because, after all, they did call me Fat-Fierce in high school!

My emotional reactions are still sometimes extreme and can cause problems in a managerial position. This is the first position I've held since graduation and it may have been a poor choice. Working in a busy, large hospital environment is not a good fit for me, although I must be doing something right. I have been doing the job for three years, received one promotion and four raises.

Besides holding a good position at SFMC, I attempt to manage a Jazz band and I also run my own business doing medical records consulting for nursing homes.

One particular morning, not long ago, on November 8, 1994, I got up early to do some consulting without giving a thought to the significance of the day. After I left the nursing home were I was working, I decided to stop by the insurance office where my mother works to take her to lunch. I walked into my mother's office and she beamed up at me from her desk. She said, "David, do you know what today is?"

A decade ago…

Thank You !

We hope you were inspired by reading *Surviving Black Ice*. Proceeds from the sale of *Surviving Black Ice* are donated to the National Brain Injury Association.

At Writer's Block Press, we are dedicated to helping our readers to recognize and reach their unimagined potential. If you have questions, comments, or insights they are welcomed…

Namaste my friends.

Please contact us at:

Writer's Block Press

PO Box 932

Killingworth, CT 06419

Or email us at:

wbpress2000@aol.com

Printed in the United States
203478BV00002B/148-195/A

9 780971 896802